WHEAT
BELLY
SLIM
GUIDE

WHEAT BELLY SLIM GUIDE

The Fast and Easy Reference
for Living and Succeeding on
the Wheat Belly Lifestyle

William Davis, MD

Author of #1 *New York Times* bestseller
Wheat Belly and *Wheat Belly Total Health*

RODALE.

RODALE *wellness*

Live happy. Be healthy. Get inspired.

Sign up today to get exclusive access to our authors, exclusive bonuses, and the most authoritative, useful, and cutting-edge information on health, wellness, fitness, and living your life to the fullest.

Visit us online at RodaleWellness.com
Join us at RodaleWellness.com/Join

© 2016 by William Davis, MD

All rights reserved. No part of this publication may be reproduced or transmitted in any form or by any means, electronic or mechanical, including photocopying, recording, or any other information storage and retrieval system, without the written permission of the publisher.

Rodale books may be purchased for business or promotional use or for special sales. For information, please write to: Special Markets Department, Rodale Inc., 733 Third Avenue, New York, NY 10017.

Printed in the United States of America
Rodale Inc. makes every effort to use acid-free ♾, recycled paper ♻.

Book design by Amy King

Library of Congress Cataloging-in-Publication Data is on file with the publisher.
ISBN 978–1–62336–854–8 paperback

Distributed to the trade by Macmillan
2 4 6 8 10 9 7 5 3 1 paperback

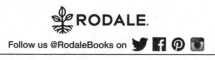

Follow us @RodaleBooks on 🐦 📘 📌 📷

We inspire health, healing, happiness, and love in the world.
Starting with you.

CONTENTS

INTRODUCTION

BAM!

What's that noise? That's the sound of the lid slamming shut on your old wheat- and grain-consuming lifestyle, the one that left you with unexplained fatigue, acid reflux, joint pain, skin rashes, headaches, constipation or bowel urgency, or even health conditions like rheumatoid arthritis or ulcerative colitis. The cut-your-fat, eat more "healthy whole grain" lifestyle you thought would provide the key to health and a size 4 bathing suit let you down, instead leading you down the path of increasing weight, expanding waistline and/or butt size, and shopping in progressively larger-size dress aisles—while your doctor, urging you to cut fat even more and pile on the grains, chastised you for your high cholesterol, high blood sugars, and high blood pressure. But funny how the doctor didn't look all that healthy or trim, nor did the office staff.

If you are new to this world of *Wheat Belly*, you may have stumbled your way into a lifestyle that transforms life and appearance by bucking all the conventional "rules" of diet, while achieving weight loss and health with an ease, rapidity, and level of success that you may have thought impossible.

More than anything else, despite rejecting all conventional rules of diet, the Wheat Belly lifestyle restores health. Yes, it would be nice to fit back into single-digit size clothes and receive envious looks from people around you who wonder why you look so vibrant, slender, and 10 years younger than your age. But wouldn't it be even better to reverse numerous common health conditions along with regaining a slender figure? That is the message of *Wheat Belly* that has turned the world of nutrition topsy-turvy, decimating decades of misguided dietary advice while restoring slender figures and health on an unprecedented scale. Yes, it may be radical, but it works. And it works big-time.

If you are already a follower of the Wheat Belly lifestyle, then this *Wheat Belly Slim Guide* can serve as a handy, portable reference at the supermarket, at restaurants, or while traveling or as a reminder of the strategies we use in the program. While you may already know that the first essential step—elimination of all wheat and grains—is readily accomplished, you also have likely come to recognize that the world is not yet set up to help you succeed. In fact, it can almost seem like it is set up for you to *fail*—thus this guide to help you get it right.

Whether you are just a few weeks into your Wheat Belly experience or you're a seasoned Wheat Belly veteran, let's briefly review what this lifestyle is all about. For the sake of size and portability, these are the essentials, some handy tools, but not the full story about why this lifestyle works so incredibly well. If you desire a better understanding of why this lifestyle packs such a huge health punch, as well as additional strategies and recipes to help you satisfy family, holiday, and entertaining needs, you will find plenty of information and resources in the *Wheat Belly* series of books and cookbooks. Visit rodalestore.com for more information on these books.

Let's put that aside for the moment—as the lid has closed, and it's getting awfully stuffy in here—and go on to a quick summary of the Wheat Belly lifestyle, seed by seed.

WHAT IS WHEAT BELLY ALL ABOUT? PLANTING THE "SEEDS" OF HEALTH

What is this talk of "seeds"?

That's what grains are: the seeds of grasses. Someone has to cut the grass on your lawn once a week or so throughout the summer. Surely, you save the nice pile of green clippings that must be good for you, right? Add some tomatoes and onions to them, then drizzle with balsamic vinaigrette—wait. You mean you *can't* eat the grass clippings? Well, why not? It's a plant, it's green, not that different from spinach, kale, or dandelion greens.

It is different because it's grass, something foreign to the human dietary experience until we made the mistake of consuming ancient grains—the seeds of grass plants—many years ago. Even ancient humans suffered a downturn in health. There was an explosion of tooth decay, iron deficiency, behavioral difficulties, and skin rashes, but they ate anything to survive, and seeds of grasses were initially a food of desperation. Bad enough in its original form, wheat and grains were made much worse by modern agribusiness when they introduced extensive genetic changes. You see the results around you, in every supermarket, school, business, and mall.

We now live in a world of plenty. Go to any supermarket and there are no shortages of food, no empty shelves, and certainly no shoppers looking emaciated and hungry. Instead, we have the opposite: shelves piled high with food and people looking like they stuff themselves silly three or more meals a day. Grains—the seeds of grasses—are no longer the food of the desperate when nothing else is available.

Ironically, misinterpretations and bad science misled us to believe that not only are grains *not* harmful, but they should serve as the cornerstone of diet—"eat more healthy whole grains"—filling breakfast, lunch, dinner, and snacks 7 days a week. If your child brings a lunch to school without a grain product, the teacher can send the lunch back home uneaten, replacing it with a grain-containing lunch instead. A modern dinner seems incomplete without buttered rolls and breaded meats, finished off with a slice of cake or pie, perhaps even accompanied by a beer—or four. Yes, the seeds of grasses have infiltrated modern habits to a degree that is unprecedented in human history, and we have paid a health price for this peculiar situation.

Genetics research and agribusiness made the situation worse because, in the interests of increasing yield-per-acre and resistance to pests, as well as other agricultural concerns, they inadvertently amplified the adverse health effects of wheat and related grains. For example, wheat germ agglutinin is a protein found in wheat, rye, barley, and rice. It is a potent bowel toxin in humans, blocking proper digestion, inflicting damage to the intestinal lining, and provoking inflammation. Genetic manipulation increased the content of wheat germ agglutinin in modern grains because it provides resistance to pests. But more pest-resistant grains means more destructive grains when we consume them. This is just one example among *dozens* of other genetic manipulations that have increased the toxic effects of grains. (A widely held misconception is that the gluten protein is the only problem with wheat and related grains, but that is far from the truth. Wheat and grains harbor *an entire collection of toxic compounds* that impair human health.)

Accept this basic fact—that humans made a mistake by incorporating the seeds of grasses into diet, a mistake made worse by modern genetic manipulations—then correct this mistake by removing all wheat and grains from your diet. When you do, unexpected and powerful changes in your health will unfold. And they will unfold in a very short time, even within the first few *days* of undertaking this lifestyle. But the effort cannot be made just 90 percent of the time, 6 days out of 7; it must be total and complete, 100 percent, with no shortcuts or corners cut, else your results will be compromised, often dramatically.

In your quest to eliminate all wheat and grains from your diet, you must therefore eliminate all obvious sources. Beyond wheat—the worst and most popular of all—this includes rye, barley, corn (yes, corn is a seed of a grass, too), oats, rice, sorghum, millet, triticale, bulgur, spelt, and kamut. Grains are promiscuous and often mate freely with each other, thereby sharing genetic traits. This means that the effects of wheat can be mimicked by rye, copied by corn, and even be revisited with a bowl of organic, no-sugar-added oatmeal. It's more or less all the same, thus the 100 percent unadulterated, no-holds-barred, complete elimination of *all* grains in the Wheat Belly lifestyle.

In case you are embarking on this grain-free journey for the first time, there are some curious phenomena that you need to be aware of. During the first week, you may feel awful: headaches, fatigue, nausea, depression. This is because wheat and grains contain a protein that is partially digested to a collection of opiates, not too different from morphine. Because you have been consuming this source of opiates for 20, 30, 40, or more years, when you remove it from your diet, you will experience an *opiate withdrawal syndrome*. It can be distinctly unpleasant for that first week, but everyone survives. Get through it and the life transformation you have dreamed of will begin, pure and simple.

Another peculiarity: Once you are grain-free for at least several weeks, any reexposure—whether intentional ("I had to have a bite of my daughter's birthday cake!") or inadvertent (sauce, roux, breading, trying to be polite at a neighborhood picnic)—can trigger a flood of awful feelings: nausea, bloating, diarrhea, dark moods or anger, joint pain, and a recurrence of any symptoms you had prior to your grain-free experience, such as migraine headaches, psoriasis, or leg edema. It is simply *not* worth it: once grain-free, always grain-free, or else you will be reminded why you undertook this lifestyle in the first place.

You are undoing a mistake that we have made as a society. Once you do so, you will reap huge and unexpected rewards in health and weight. Stick with it and wonderful changes are in your future.

SOMEWHERE OVER THE RAINBOW

In the Wheat Belly lifestyle, we do *not* count calories, push the plate away, or eat smaller portions. We are eliminating a group of foods that were never suited to be foods in the first place, no matter how tasty or pretty they were made to be by clever but unsuspecting humans. Remove this dietary toxin and you can finally start on the path to effortless weight loss, clear your mind of mind "fog," be released from an extraordinary list of aches and pains, reduce or completely disable inflammation, normalize hormonal distortions, be freed from acid reflux and the bowel urgency or constipation of irritable bowel syndrome, drop blood sugars dramatically, and reduce or be entirely freed from prescription medications.

Dreams really do come true in this lifestyle, all achieved by doing the *opposite* of what all conventional dietary advice has been telling you for years.

CHAPTER 1

HOW TO USE THIS *SLIM GUIDE*

WHEAT BELLY SLIM GUIDE is meant to be a handy, portable resource to carry with you while shopping, eating at restaurants, or navigating other situations outside the home. It can also serve as a quick reminder of the concepts discussed in the *Wheat Belly* books, including the additional strategies covered in *Wheat Belly Total Health* and *Wheat Belly 10-Day Grain Detox* that stack the odds in favor of reversing numerous health conditions, from type 2 diabetes to eczema to ulcerative colitis.

In this guide, you will find a summary of the main points in the Wheat Belly lifestyle, the nutritional supplements we include, how to choose an effective probiotic, your choices in prebiotic fibers, a grocery shopping list, a list of hidden sources of wheat and corn in processed foods, and our choices of safe flours for baking, as well as safe sweeteners and thickeners. You will also find some of the most popular recipes among readers of the *Wheat Belly* cookbooks woven into a 7-day sample menu plan, along with other popular recipes taken from these cookbooks, and a listing of safe alcoholic beverages. I've included several discussions to help keep you on course, such as the top 10 reasons why we eliminate all wheat and grains, common mistakes to avoid, what to do when you experience food cravings, and how to eat safely when eating outside the home.

You will be reminded that, by living the Wheat Belly lifestyle, we reject nearly all conventional dietary rules. We do not limit fat or saturated fat, never count calories, thumb our noses at cholesterol, and throw notions of moderation, "balance," and various pyramids and plates into the trash. The last 50 years have been a dietary dead end for Americans, evidenced during any visit to the mall or grocery store by people overweight and unhealthy on a scale never before witnessed. We are no longer going to play that game.

Add it all up and this guide is designed to help you succeed in ways you never anticipated, on a scale you never thought possible. Clear your bookshelves of all the books preaching calorie cutting, fat reduction, moderation, and all the other misery-yielding, tortured advice that is unnatural and unproductive. Let's instead engage in a program that is natural and tasty and simply works. The Wheat Belly lifestyle is a life-changing experience, and this guide can help you achieve it.

CHAPTER 2

THE TOP 10 REASONS TO KICK ALL WHEAT AND GRAINS OUT OF YOUR LIFE

ALTHOUGH WE ARE told over and over again that "healthy whole grains" should be a staple in every meal, every day there are plenty of reasons to never allow your lips to meet a wheat bagel, a sandwich, or pretzels again. Banishing all wheat and grains from your diet is among the most powerful health strategies you can adopt.

But, because we are barraged with the "healthy whole grain" message every day from TV, magazines, and even the government, friends and neighbors will inevitably ask you *why* you have chosen to engage in such a contrary lifestyle. This list of the Top 10 Reasons to Kick All Wheat and Grains Out of Your Life will keep the most important reasons on the tip of your tongue. (If you want even more details on why and how the Wheat Belly lifestyle provides such a powerful path to health and weight loss, see the *Wheat Belly* books, especially *Wheat Belly Total Health*.)

The top 10 reasons why wheat and grains should never be consumed by humans are:

1. Gliadin is a protein in wheat, rye, and barley that, upon partial digestion, yields opiates that bind to the brain's opiate receptors and *increase appetite*. This is a big part of the reason that grains make you suffer with continual hunger, make you gain weight, and can trigger addictive relationships with foods like pizza and cookies.

2. Gliadin-derived opiates behave like mind-active drugs that trigger behavioral outbursts in kids with attention-deficit disorder and autism, paranoia in people with schizophrenia, depression in susceptible people, and 24-hour-a-day food obsessions in people prone to bulimia and binge-eating disorder.

3. Gliadin increases intestinal permeability and initiates the process of autoimmunity leading to rheumatoid arthritis, type 1 diabetes, multiple sclerosis, psoriasis, and 200 other conditions.

4. Amylopectin A, the "complex" carbohydrate of grains, raises blood sugar higher, ounce for ounce, than table sugar. Eating plenty of "healthy whole grains" at each meal ensures high blood sugars every time you do so, taking you closer to type 2 diabetes.

5. Wheat germ agglutinin is a potent bowel toxin among several others in wheat and grains that lead to acid

reflux, irritable bowel syndrome, and other gastrointestinal conditions, as well as body-wide inflammation due to the small quantities that gain entry into the bloodstream via the increased intestinal permeability initiated by the gliadin protein.

6. Wheat germ agglutinin blocks gallbladder and pancreatic function (by blocking the receptor for the digestive hormone, cholecystokinin), adding further to digestive difficulties, constipation, and dysbiosis (unhealthy changes in bowel microorganisms that impact health in many ways).

7. Grain phytates block absorption of minerals such as iron, zinc, calcium, and magnesium. Many cases of unexplained iron deficiency anemia, for instance— severe enough to be "treated" with blood transfusions— reverse within several weeks of eliminating grains.

8. Multiple allergenic proteins are present, such as trypsin inhibitors, thioreductases, alpha-amylase inhibitors, and gamma gliadins—responsible for asthma, skin rashes, and gastrointestinal distress.

9. Grains are potent endocrine disrupters, explaining why women with polycystic ovarian syndrome are much worse with grain consumption; why men grow breasts along with belly fat; why male levels of testosterone drop and estrogen increases; why cortisol action is blocked, resulting in fatigue; and why thyroid health is disrupted by autoimmune inflammation.

10. Big Food and agribusiness use wheat and grains to control human buying behavior, putting the addictive appetite-stimulating effects of wheat and grains to work by increasing food consumption to keep you coming back for more.

Most people do not realize that grains are the seeds of grasses and that humans are digestively ill equipped to consume any part of grass plants, including the seeds. Many of the problems with grains originate with indigestible or poorly digestible proteins. Wheat germ agglutinin, for example, is entirely resistant to human digestion but exerts all manner of odd gastrointestinal inflammatory and hormonally disruptive effects in its passage from mouth to toilet. Gliadin, if left intact, initiates the autoimmune processed described above, but it can also be partially digested to peptides—not single amino acids like other proteins—that have unique amino acid sequences that allow binding to opiate receptors of the human brain. The exception to the poor digestibility of the seeds of grasses is amylopectin A, the carbohydrate that accounts for the exceptional blood sugar–raising potential of grains.

Minus the appetite-stimulating, health-disrupting effects of the various components of grains, you are back in the driver's seat for controlling appetite, weight, and health.

CHAPTER 3

THE BASIC RULES OF LIVING THE WHEAT BELLY LIFESTYLE

GET THE BASICS of the Wheat Belly lifestyle right, and incredible things can happen in short order: dramatic weight loss without limiting calories, reduced appetite and freedom from cravings, freedom from joint pain, reversal of acid reflux and irritable bowel syndrome symptoms, and reduction or outright reversal of serious conditions such as rheumatoid arthritis and other autoimmune diseases and type 2 diabetes.

Inflammation typically starts receding within the first few days, changes that can be evidenced by a reduction in facial puffiness and loss of around-the-eye circles and puffiness, even making your eyes seem larger—changes that go beyond just weight loss. Cutting calories does not reverse inflammation; removing the foods that cause inflammation reverses it. Yes, get the Wheat Belly lifestyle right and you can achieve far more than you ever thought possible, more than any calorie-cutting or exercise program could accomplish, while minimizing or eliminating your need for prescription drugs.

But get it wrong just by a little bit and success can be completely blocked. This is because the effects of the wrong choices in foods can be so overpowering that they even negate the benefits of healthy choices. So let's go over the basic rules of living the Wheat Belly lifestyle, the essential details that we all follow to return to a state of ideal health and weight.

Note that the Wheat Belly lifestyle begins with the most crucial step of all—elimination of all wheat and grains—but it does not end there. Several additional steps are necessary to correct deficiencies/abnormalities created by long-term grain consumption as well as some common deficiencies shared by most people that can obstruct your success. (See Chapter 4, Beyond the Wheat Belly Way of Eating.)

The Wheat Belly lifestyle therefore begins with several simple dietary rules to help you avoid problem foods while helping you make good choices, condensed into a three-step process:

Step 1:   Eliminate all grains.

Step 2:   Choose real, single-ingredient foods.

Step 3:   Manage carbohydrates.

STEP 1: ELIMINATE ALL GRAINS

We start by eliminating the unexpected and surprising source of so many problems: no, not your spouse's excessive sports TV-watching habits, but grains. It is not uncommon for people to obtain more than *half* of their daily calories from grains. Eliminating them therefore represents a major disruption of shopping, eating, and cooking habits. But I know of nothing else—exercise, prescription drugs, nutritional supplements, meditation, cleansing enemas, a year in a monastery—that can match the benefits of removing these disrupters of health.

This first step is therefore unavoidable. You *cannot* succeed in this lifestyle without this critical first step; none of the other steps will follow nor will you achieve the effects you desire. So don't skimp on this step; follow it 100 percent.

Start by Purging Your Kitchen of All Grains

Start this lifestyle by creating a grain-free kitchen: your refrigerator, pantry, and cabinet shelves should be free of all grains and grain-containing products.

Remember: Grains are added to bulk up a product inexpensively, causing you to believe that the $5.99 deep-dish pizza is a bargain when in fact it's just loaded with cheap filler. The dirty little secret is that grains increase food consumption by yielding opiates that increase appetite. It's not uncommon for grains to provoke consumption of 1,000 or more additional calories per day in an adult.

Yes, purging your kitchen means tossing out a lot of stuff. Throw them in the trash, give them to charity, use them for compost or cat litter—but get rid of them. This removes the temptation to "just have one cracker" or think that "just one bite won't hurt" or finish them in order to avoid waste. Making the break abruptly and cleanly is very important for your success. If you are unable to completely purge your kitchen of grain products due to, say, a spouse or other family member who refuses to go along with your lifestyle change, make it clear that you are going to have food set aside to suit your new eating choices.

Start by removing all obvious sources of wheat flour such as breads, rolls, doughnuts, pasta, cookies, cakes, pretzels, crackers, pancake mix, breakfast cereals, bread crumbs, and bagels. Then remove all bottled, canned, packaged, and frozen processed foods with wheat among the ingredients. Check the labels for wheat in all its various forms, some of which are obvious and others that are not, with names such as modified food starch, panko, seitan, and bran. (See Chapter 17 for a listing of hidden grain sources.)

Tackle barley-containing foods next. This includes any food with "malt" listed on the label, as well as barley itself. Beer and some other alcoholic beverages (see Chapter 12) should go, as well as any foods made with rye, such as rye breads and rye crackers.

Then remove all obvious sources of **corn**, such as corn on the cob, canned corn, corn chips, tacos, and grits. As with wheat, also remove processed foods made with not-so-obvious corn ingredients such as hydrolyzed cornstarch and polenta (also listed in Chapter 17).

Other grains, such as oats, rice, millet, sorghum, amaranth, and teff, are usually listed by their real names; purge the kitchen of these foods, too. (Don't be fooled by their lack of gluten: They still raise blood sugar sky-high, blocking all hopes of losing weight or regaining full health.)

Start Your Grain-Free Wheat Belly Lifestyle

1. Clearing your kitchen of all obvious grain wheat and grain sources, as follows:

Wheat-based products: bread, rolls, hot and cold breakfast cereals, noodles, pasta, bagels, muffins, pancakes and pancake mixes, waffles, doughnuts, pretzels, cookies, crackers, orzo, bread crumbs

Bulgur and triticale (both related to wheat)

Barley products: barley, barley breads, soups with barley, vinegars with barley malt

Rye products: rye bread, pumpernickel bread, crackers

Corn products: corn, cornstarch, cornmeal products (chips, tacos, tortillas), grits, polenta, sauces or gravies thickened with cornstarch, corn syrup, high-fructose corn syrup, breakfast cereals

Rice products: white rice, brown rice, wild rice, rice cakes, breakfast cereals

Oat products: oatmeal, oat bran, oat cereals

Amaranth

Teff

Millet

Sorghum

2. Then eliminate hidden sources by reading labels.

Eliminate hidden sources of grains by avoiding the processed foods that fill the inner aisles of the grocery store. Almost all of these foods are thickened, flavored, or textured with grain products or contain grains added as cheap filler. Living without grains means avoiding foods that you never thought contained grains, such as seasoning mixes bulked up with cornstarch, canned and dry soup mixes with wheat flour, Twizzlers, granola bars, soy sauce, frozen dinners with wheat-containing gravy, and muffins.

Go Grain-Free Shopping

You've purged your kitchen of grain-containing foods and need to restock with new, healthy, grain-free alternatives. It's time to go the supermarket or the stores where you shop for meat, vegetables, and other foods.

Of the 60,000 or so processed food products that pack the shelves of the average supermarket, your options will be cut down to about 1,000, but you should *never* feel deprived. You will discover that the foods you've eliminated are nearly all variations on the same processed food themes: wheat flour, cornstarch, sugar, high-fructose corn syrup, and food coloring whether it was labeled breakfast cereal, a pop-in-the-toaster convenience breakfast, low-calorie frozen dinners, or crackers, all cheap filler dolled up with the glitz of modern marketing.

Start by *not* shopping for obvious sources of wheat, corn, and other grains. Avoid the bread aisle, the bakery, frozen food freezers, the breakfast cereal aisle, and the internal aisles stocked with packaged foods. Confine your shopping to the produce section, the butcher counter, and the dairy refrigerator; venture into the inner aisles only for spices, nuts and seeds, laundry detergent and other household supplies, and pet food. (Consult the shopping list in Chapter 11 to be sure you've got the ingredients on hand to create dishes that fit into the Wheat Belly lifestyle and that you will need to follow Wheat Belly recipes and the 7-day menu plan.)

You are aiming to achieve a diet filled with foods that are least processed. Choose foods that are *naturally* grain-free, such as vegetables, eggs, olives, and meats. That points us toward another rule that helps you navigate your new life: Avoid processed foods that bear labels and return to real, single-ingredient foods without labels. Minus the processed foods that fill supermarket shelves, we return to unprocessed, naturally grain-free foods.

STEP 2: CHOOSE REAL, SINGLE-INGREDIENT FOODS

No food manufacturer adds grains to an avocado or eggs in their shell. Foods left intact and unmodified by a food manufacturer should top your list of foods to choose that are safe. Avocados and whole eggs are real and chance no exposure to grains, added sugars, high-fructose corn syrup, hydrogenated oils, or other no-no's.

You will find the majority of real, single-ingredient foods in the produce section, butcher counter, and dairy refrigerator. Depending on the layout of your supermarket, you may have to venture into hazardous internal aisles for some of your baking supplies, spices, and nuts, but do so while ignoring all the processed, glitzy, eye-catching products. Ignore the sales, the samples being offered, and all the tricks used to capture attention such as cartoon characters or sports figures.

Avoiding foods with labels simplifies the task of label reading. Cucumbers, spinach, and pork chops, for example, don't come with labels (except to display weight and date).

Avoiding labels means you'll be buying foods in their basic, least modified forms.

Choosing real, single-ingredient foods means enjoying unlimited quantities of:

BEVERAGES—Drink water (squeeze in some lemon or lime, or keep a filled water pitcher in the refrigerator with a few slices of cucumber, kiwi, or orange or mint leaves), teas (black, green, or white), infusions (teas brewed from other leaves, herbs, flowers, and fruits), unsweetened almond milk, unsweetened coconut milk (carton variety from the dairy refrigerator), unsweetened hemp milk, and coffee. Avoid sodas and fruit drinks, even if the soda is sugar-free, since sugar-free beverages are typically sweetened with aspartame, acesulfame, saccharine, or sucralose and have been associated with weight gain and unhealthy changes in bowel flora that encourage diabetes.

CHEESES—Eat real cultured cheeses only (not Velveeta or single-slice processed cheese), preferably organic and full-fat, not skim or reduced-fat. The cheese-making process minimizes the undesirable aspects of dairy (such as whey and unhealthy forms of casein). Be careful with blue cheese, Gorgonzola, and Roquefort, which are occasionally sources of wheat.

EGGS—Eggs are little powerhouses of nutrition and are an important part of a successful grain-free lifestyle. We do not limit eggs. Choose cage-free or pastured, organic sources whenever possible; even better, purchase them from a local source. If you are allergic to eggs from chickens, consider goose, duck, ostrich, or quail eggs, whenever available.

FATS AND OILS—Choose coconut, extra-virgin olive, extra-light olive, macadamia, avocado, and walnut oils, as well as organic butter and ghee. Don't be afraid of saving the lard and tallow from bacon, beef, and pork. Or purchase lard and tallow from the grocery, but check to be sure they are not hydrogenated. Don't overdo polyunsaturated oils (corn, safflower, mixed vegetable, and sunflower) and ignore any claims of "heart healthy" (which is entirely untrue). Avoid hydrogenated or partially hydrogenated oils completely.

MEATS—Beef, pork, lamb, fish, chicken, turkey, buffalo, and ostrich should be pastured/grass-fed, free-range, and organic whenever possible to minimize antibiotic residues and hormones. Choose fatty cuts, often less expensive and full of the fats you need. Try to overcome the modern aversion to organ meats, such as liver, heart, and tongue, the most nutritious components of all (especially liver and heart). Uncured liver sausage or ground liver added to meat loaf is an easy way to jump-start organ consumption. Save bones in the freezer to make soups and stocks, excellent for joint, hair, and nail health.

OTHER FOODS—Guacamole, hummus, unsweetened condiments (e.g., mayonnaise, mustard, oil-based salad dressings without high-fructose corn syrup, sugar, dextrose, or cornstarch), ketchup without high-fructose corn syrup, pesto, tapenades, and olives are all good to have on hand.

RAW OR DRY-ROASTED NUTS AND SEEDS—Almonds, walnuts, pecans, hazelnuts, pistachios, Brazil nuts, macadamias, pumpkin seeds, sunflower seeds, sesame seeds, flaxseeds, and chia seeds are all great choices, as are dry-roasted peanuts (not really a nut, but a low-carbohydrate legume). Avoid nuts roasted in unhealthy oils, such as hydrogenated cottonseed or hydrogenated soybean oil, as well as wheat flour, cornstarch, maltodextrin, or sugar used to coat them. Cashews are an exception, as they are carbohydrate-heavy; consume lightly and use the carbohydrate management method discussed in Step 3.

VEGETABLES—Enjoy all the fresh or frozen veggies you want, except for potatoes (which we only consume raw). Explore the wonderful range of choices: spinach, chard, kale, broccoli, broccolini, collard greens, lettuces, peppers, onions, mushrooms, Brussels sprouts, zucchini, squash, and so on. Keep in mind that people undergo a dramatic change in taste perception upon going grain-free, so it may be time to revisit vegetables you didn't previously enjoy. Don't be surprised if the Brussels sprouts you once despised soon become your favorite. Minimize reliance on canned vegetables, especially tomatoes, due to bisphenol A, an endocrine-disrupting chemical, in the can's resin lining.

Stock Your Kitchen with Real, Whole Foods

BEVERAGES—Teas, coffee, infusions (teas brewed from other leaves, herbs, flowers, and fruits), unsweetened almond milk, unsweetened coconut milk (carton variety from the dairy refrigerator), unsweetened hemp milk

CHEESE—Real, full-fat, cultured cheeses only, preferably organic

EGGS—Cage-free or pastured, organic, and purchased from a local source

FATS AND OILS—Coconut, extra-virgin olive, extra-light olive, macadamia, avocado, walnut, organic butter and ghee, lard and tallow from bacon, beef, and pork (nonhydrogenated if purchased)

MEATS—Beef, pork, lamb, fish, chicken, turkey, buffalo, ostrich. Choose meats that are pastured/grass-fed, free-range, and from organic sources whenever possible. Choose fattier, never lean, cuts.

OTHER FOODS—Guacamole, hummus, unsweetened condiments (e.g., mayonnaise, mustard, oil-based salad dressings without high-fructose corn syrup, sugar, dextrose, or cornstarch), ketchup without high-fructose corn syrup, pesto, tapenades, olives

RAW OR DRY-ROASTED NUTS AND SEEDS—Almonds, walnuts, pecans, hazelnuts, pistachios, Brazil nuts, macadamias, dry-roasted peanuts, pumpkin seeds, sunflower seeds, sesame seeds, flaxseeds, chia seeds

VEGETABLES—Spinach, chard, kale, broccoli, broccolini, collard greens, cucumbers, lettuces, peppers, onions, mushrooms, Brussels sprouts, zucchini, squash, etc. (We do include white potatoes, but eat them raw for their prebiotic fiber benefits.)

STEP 3: MANAGE CARBOHYDRATES

There are very few things we count in the Wheat Belly life-style. We *never* count calories or fat grams, for instance. Nor do we engage in elaborate swap systems or track points, and we do not point you toward costly, highly processed protein pow-der meal replacements. But, because so many people hope to lose weight and/or are struggling with blood sugar issues or insulin resistance, we do count one value: carbohydrate grams. Carbohydrates mess with blood sugar and insulin and thereby slow, or completely block, weight loss and health efforts. Get-ting this part of the Wheat Belly lifestyle right will help you lose weight faster and regain health more confidently. And it will give you further control over fatty liver, triglycerides, blood pressure, and needing to shop in plus-size aisles, adding further firepower to even the most meticulous grain-free start. This step is also necessary to take control over the modern epidemics of type 2 diabetes and prediabetes, or just the insulin resistance that is the rule in modern people, and sets you up for future health struggles.

The third step in preparing to live your new Wheat Belly–empowered life is therefore to manage carbohydrates, the dar-lings of the processed food industry and cheap, tasty fillers that contribute to dietary helplessness and health distortions.

It's not total carbohydrates that matter, but what are called net carbohydrates. Fiber, though counted as a carbohydrate in nutrition fact tables, is not metabolized to blood sugar, and we can therefore subtract it from the total to yield net carbohydrates.

We follow this simple rule: **Never exceed 15 grams (g) of net carbohydrates per meal**. This is a very important value to follow. To calculate net carbs:

NET CARBS = TOTAL CARBS—FIBER

To find the carb and fiber composition of various foods, you will need a resource such as an inexpensive handbook with tables of the nutritional content of foods (found in the reference section of the bookstore or library, often for less than $10). There are smartphone apps useful for this purpose. (Search for "nutritional analysis" in your application source. Nutrition Lookup by SparkPeople and Food Facts by FatSecret Platform API are two popular choices, downloadable for free.) There are also Web sites such as NutritionData (www.nutritiondata.com) that list nutritional analyses of foods.

Look up total carbohydrate and fiber content of the food in question, make the simple calculation, and you'll have net carbohydrate content. (But ignore all advice about ways to cut calories, fat grams, portion sizes—all the advice we ignore in our grain-free and empowered Wheat Belly lifestyle.)

For example, to calculate net carbs for a medium-size Red Delicious apple, look up total carbs and fiber:

Total carbs: 22.0 g, fiber: 5.0 g. Calculate net carbs by the equation:

22.0 G—5.0 G = 17.0 G NET CARBS

This exceeds our 15 g net carb cutoff, just enough to stall weight-loss efforts and raise blood sugar modestly. So eat only half an apple or buy smaller apples.

To help you stick to this guideline, choose fruit with the lowest carbohydrate content and greatest nutritional value. From best to worst, choose from: berries of all varieties, cherries, citrus, apples, nectarines, peaches, and melons. One-half cup of blueberries, for example, contains 15 g total carbohydrates and 3 g fiber, which equals 12 g net carbohydrates. This easily fits into your 15 g net carbs or less. Minimize ripe bananas, pineapples, mangoes, and grapes—eat them only in small quantities, since their sugar content is similar to that of candy. A ripe 7-inch banana, for example, contains 27 g total carbohydrates and 3 g fiber: 27 - 3 = 24 g net carbohydrates. That's enough to turn off weight loss and trigger weight *gain* (but we do include green unripe bananas for their prebiotic fiber content and, if truly green, *zero* net carb content). An exception to fruit guidelines is avocados, which are high in fats, rich in potassium, wonderfully filling, and low in net carbs (3 g per avocado), as close to a perfect fruit as you can get.

Net carb calculations are not necessary for foods such as meats, poultry, fish, eggs, green vegetables, mushrooms, coconut oil, butter, or full-fat cheeses. But calculations will be necessary for starchy vegetables and legumes, fruits (except avocados), other dairy products, nuts, and seeds.

Don't be thrown off course by following the misleading concept of the glycemic index or glycemic load. Choosing low-glycemic index foods, for instance, will trigger blood sugar and insulin to high levels, cause weight gain, and prevent the health benefits of this lifestyle—virtually no different than high-glycemic index foods. Do not fall for the health and weight booby trap of glycemic index, an entirely useless concept.

You will find that, after calculating net carbs for a handful of foods, you'll quickly get the hang of it and know which foods are safe and which are not, without even having to perform the calculation. (You will also notice that many low-glycemic and medium-glycemic index foods exceed our carb cutoff by a wide margin, explaining why even low-glycemic index foods turn off your ability to lose weight and regain full control over health.) You will identify what foods and how much fit into your lifestyle, while also realizing that you can consume unlimited amounts of foods with zero or low net carb counts.

Do *Not* Limit Fats!

It is important that, as part of your carbohydrate management effort, you *do not limit fats or oils*. In the Wheat Belly lifestyle, there are no limits on fat or oil intake, provided you choose your sources wisely. It means you should enjoy fat on meats. Don't buy lean meats, buy fatty cuts. Don't trim fat off beef, pork, lamb, or poultry—eat it. Save fats from cooking beef, pork, and bacon in a glass container and refrigerate to use as cooking oil. Save the bones (or buy from a butcher) to make soup or stock, and don't skim off the fat when it cools. Don't limit egg consumption; have a three-egg omelet, for instance, with lots of extra-virgin olive oil, pesto, or olive oil–soaked sun-dried tomatoes. Use the oils listed above generously in every dish possible.

If you are worried about your cholesterol, know that the majority of people will experience a *reduction* in LDL ("bad") cholesterol with this lifestyle, along with plummeting triglycerides and a rise in healthy HDL. Eating fats and oils normalizes these predictors of cardiovascular risk. (You can find a full discussion of the *why* behind these unexpected changes, and why and how a low-fat diet ruins health and increases cardiovascular risk, in both the original *Wheat Belly* and in *Wheat Belly Total Health*.)

We avoid all foods labeled "low-fat" and "nonfat." These terms mean high-carbohydrate and added sugars or high-fructose corn syrup. If you consume dairy products, pour the skim or 2% milk down the drain and go for full-fat or cream. And no "light" coconut milk—we want the thickest, fattiest variety.

We do, however, avoid all hydrogenated ("trans") fats, a common ingredient in processed foods, especially grain-based foods, as they contribute to heart disease, hypertension, and diabetes. Margarine is the worst, made with vegetable oils hydrogenated to yield a solid stick or tub form. Many processed foods, from cookies to sandwich spreads, contain hydrogenated oils and should be avoided for this and other reasons. Use real organic butter or ghee instead (if you include dairy).

Despite our embrace of fats and oils, do not interpret this to mean that foods deep-fried in oils are healthy. They are not. It's not the fat that's the problem, but the high-temperature reactions that occur in deep-fried foods. These reactions result in health-impairing by-products, so we minimize or avoid foods that are deep-fried.

We Do NOT Include Gluten-Free Processed Foods!

Gluten-free foods made with cornstarch, rice flour, tapioca starch, or potato flour are not included in the Wheat Belly lifestyle. These are the four ingredients most commonly found in gluten-free processed foods. They are awful for health and will completely shut down any hope of weight loss, often resulting in weight *gain* and inflammation.

Managing carbohydrates means 100 percent avoidance of these awful products marketed to an unsuspecting public thinking they are eating healthy by avoiding "gluten." *Nothing* raises blood sugar higher than the gluten-free junk carbohydrates in, say, gluten-free multigrain bread or gluten-free pasta—higher than even table sugar.

Think of the Wheat Belly lifestyle as being *grain*-free, not gluten-free—a much safer, more effective path. (Ironically, many people who have heard of the powerful Wheat Belly message but have not read the books presume that it is nothing more than a gluten-free lifestyle filled with gluten-free replacement foods. You now know that is the farthest thing from the truth. The Wheat Belly lifestyle *rejects* all such health-impairing, obesity-causing gluten-free foods.)

There are some food producers who have developed gluten-free and grain-free products without junk carb ingredients that do not raise blood sugar and are therefore safe. But they remain in the minority.

A FEW ADDITIONAL RULES FOR CHOOSING FOODS FOR YOUR WHEAT BELLY LIFESTYLE

In addition to choosing real, single-ingredient foods, there are some other ground rules to know that will help you choose genuinely healthy foods at the grocery.

MEATS SHOULD NOT BE CURED WITH SODIUM NITRITE. Sausage, pepperoni, bacon, salami, and other processed meats often contain the color-fixing preservative sodium nitrite. Upon cooking, sodium nitrite reacts with amino acids in meat, yielding nitrosamines that have been linked to gastrointestinal cancers. Look for meats labeled "uncured" and without sodium nitrite listed on the label (not to be confused with nitrates, which do not react to form nitrosamines). Also make sure processed meats, especially luncheon meats, sausage, and deli meats contain no wheat, cornstarch, or other hidden grains. If you cannot view the ingredient list, don't buy it.

CHOOSE ORGANIC DAIRY PRODUCTS. Minimize excess estrogen content, bovine growth hormone, and antibiotics by choosing dairy products from organic producers.

CHOOSE ORGANIC VEGETABLES AND FRUITS. Whenever available and budget permitting, make organic your first choice—most important when the exterior of the food is consumed, as with blueberries and broccoli, for example. If you cannot choose organic, at the very least rinse fruits and veggies thoroughly in warm water to minimize pesticide and herbicide residues that have been linked to cancer and endocrine disruption.

DON'T OVERLY RESTRICT SALT. Most of us engaged in a grain-free lifestyle should use mineral-rich forms of salt, such as sea salt, which is healthier than severely restricting salt, particularly when that salt is combined with healthy foods rich in potassium (such as from vegetables, avocados, or coconut). Because the first week in particular of the Wheat Belly lifestyle involves increased salt and water loss in the urine (explaining why, for instance, leg edema and facial puffiness are typically lost within the first several days), we have to compensate by an increased intake of both salt and water. For this reason, we lightly salt our food.

In fact, advice to severely restrict salt has been formally retracted in view of clinical studies demonstrating *increased* cardiovascular death with salt restriction of 1,500 mg per day or less. There can be problems, however, with unlimited salt use, as occurs with consumption of canned sodas and fast food, as salt intakes of 6,000 to 10,000 mg per day can indeed be associated with adverse cardiovascular effects. (Anyone with kidney disease, edema, or severe hypertension may develop salt sensitivity and should adhere to the sodium prescription provided by your doctor.)

CHAPTER 4

BEYOND THE WHEAT BELLY WAY OF EATING

GETTING THE DIETARY rules of the Wheat Belly way of eating right, as discussed in Chapter 3, will get you off to a powerful start. But the diet alone does not solve all problems.

For example, bowel health and the composition of bowel flora (the microorganisms in your bowels) are so disrupted by prior grain consumption (and other factors such as antibiotics and chlorinated drinking water) that removing grains alone does not allow full healing and restoration of healthy flora. Additional efforts will be needed. Absorption of minerals such as magnesium is almost completely blocked by grain consumption; everyone therefore starts with substantial magnesium deficiency. While removing grains removes the blockers (phytates) of magnesium absorption, deficiency is more rapidly corrected with supplementation. Still other nutrients, such as iodine and vitamin D, are commonly deficient in most people; though this is not caused by prior grain consumption, correction yields additional health benefits.

As with the diet we follow in the Wheat Belly lifestyle, get this part right and even more spectacular improvements can be expected in your health.

MANAGE YOUR GARDEN OF BOWEL FLORA

Add a probiotic with 30 billion to 50 billion CFUs per day and at least a dozen species

Prebiotic fibers: 10 grams (g) per day first week, 20 g per day thereafter

The organisms inhabiting your intestines are not just important but *critical* for overall health. Having a healthy, diverse profile of microorganisms in your intestines helps control weight, reduces triglycerides and blood sugar, reduces blood pressure, encourages bowel regularity, prevents colon cancer, and even influences sleep quality and mental health. When you remove grains, a major factor disrupting bowel flora has been removed. This therefore represents a wonderful opportunity to reestablish bowel flora that brings you closer to achieving your health and weight-loss goals.

It helps to view bowel flora as being like a backyard garden. To have a successful garden in springtime, you prepare the soil and plant seeds. You then need to water and fertilize your garden. This is how it works with bowel flora. We need to plant "seeds"—probiotics that contain healthy organisms—then "water and fertilize" the garden by providing prebiotic fibers that nourish preferred species over time.

We therefore start this process by "seeding" your intestines with a high-potency probiotic supplement with a "colony-forming unit," or CFU, count of at least 30 billion to 50 billion per day. It also means providing a wide diversity of species. The best probiotics typically contain a dozen or more species, such as *Lactobacillus plantarum* and *Bifidobacterium infantis*. (Garden of Life Raw and Renew Life Ultimate Flora are two excellent probiotic preparations.) You only need to take probiotics for a limited time, e.g., 6 to 8 weeks, long enough to reseed your intestines with healthy species, provided you properly nourish them. (People with chronic bowel conditions, such as Crohn's disease, ulcerative colitis, or celiac disease, typically need to take a probiotic for much longer, even years, as intestinal health recovers over a more extended time period.)

The "water and fertilizer" prebiotic fibers come from some unusual sources—underground roots and tubers extracted by digging in the dirt. Because you likely have little time or interest in digging in the forest, we choose modern equivalents of primitive sources, easy to find in stores. Don't confuse these fibers with cellulose, or wood fiber, the fiber in bran cereals and other products that provide "bulk" and yield bowel regularity; they do *not* provide nutrition to bowel microorganisms, nor do they contribute to other healthy changes in bowel flora.

During your first week of the Wheat Belly lifestyle, we aim to obtain no more than 10 g prebiotic fibers per day. After your initial week, increase your intake to a total of 20 g per day.

However, if you experience excessive gas, bloating, or discomfort when you begin your initial 10 g per day or when you increase to 20 g per day, this suggests that you have severe dysbiosis or disruption of bowel flora. Should either situation occur, stop the prebiotic fibers while continuing the probiotic; after 4 weeks of the probiotic alone, begin the prebiotic fiber process over again. If discomfort recurs, then it's time to consult *Wheat Belly Total Health* or *Wheat Belly 10-Day Grain Detox* for solutions, or discuss further with a well-informed health practitioner such as a functional medicine or integrative health practitioner (almost never a primary care doctor or gastroenterologist, who will dismiss your concerns and/or have no idea what to do).

Obtain prebiotic fibers from:

Green bananas and plantains: 11 g fiber in one medium banana. The banana must be truly green and unripe.

Raw white potato (coarsely peeled): 20 g fiber per 1 medium (3½ inches length)

Hummus: 15 g fiber in ¼ cup (10 g net carbohydrates)

Inulin and fructooligosaccharide (FOS) powders: 5 g fiber per teaspoon

Lentils: 2.5 g fiber in ½ cup (11 g net carbohydrates)

Beans: 3.8 g fiber in ½ cup—white beans are the richest with twice this quantity (12 g net carbohydrates)

The easiest way to accomplish this is to include a coarsely chopped green banana or raw potato in a smoothie every day. (You can find recipes for Detox Shakes in *Wheat Belly 10-Day Grain Detox*.) Inulin or FOS powders (found in health food stores) are an especially convenient way to obtain such fibers, added to your smoothie or other foods.

During your first week, when you are trying to obtain no more than 10 g fiber per day, only use about *half* of the green banana or *half* of the raw potato in your smoothie, or no more than 1 to 2 teaspoons of inulin/FOS; after the first week, build up to the target of 20 g per day.

I like to slice or chop a raw potato into small cubes to include in salads, add a couple of teaspoons of powdered inulin to various dishes, and dip vegetables or grain-free crackers into hummus. Consuming small quantities—no more than ¼ cup per meal—of lentils, chickpeas, and starchy beans (black, kidney, white, lima) adds to your daily total. Root vegetables (onions, sweet potatoes, parsnips, rutabaga, the Peruvian plant maca, celeriac, daikon, and others) likewise add modest quantities of a gram or two of these fibers, but just be careful to not exceed your 15 g net carbs per meal.

The benefits of this powerful strategy, such as lower blood pressure and deeper sleep, develop slowly over 2 to 3 months (or longer) as healthy species proliferate and exert their metabolic benefits body-wide, effects that compound the wonderful health changes started with wheat and grain elimination. It's a powerful synergy that adds up to some pretty darned magnificent improvements in health.

SUPPLEMENT VITAMIN D

4,000 to 8,000 international units per day as vitamin D_3 gelcaps,
best taken in the morning

Restore vitamin D to healthy levels and wonderful things happen: improved mood, clearer thinking, better bone health and protection from osteoporosis, reduced blood sugar and blood pressure, improved physical performance, protection from dementia and cancer—compounding many of the wonderful effects begun by wheat and grain elimination. Many people actually *feel* the beneficial effects of vitamin D restoration, especially improved mood and mental clarity, as well as relief from seasonal "blues." Inflammation and autoimmune conditions, such as rheumatoid arthritis and psoriasis, can improve because once the initial trigger for these conditions—wheat and grains—has been removed, restoring vitamin D further reverses the abnormal inflammatory and immune responses that allowed these diseases to manifest.

Most people achieve the target 25-hydroxy vitamin D blood level of 60 to 70 nanograms per milliliter after taking 4,000 to 8,000 units per day of oil-based vitamin D_3, or cholecalciferol (in gelcap or drops, not tablets, to ensure absorption) for 2 to 3 months. Not restricting foods such as egg yolks and liver also makes a modest contribution. Remember: Getting a lot of sun exposure and having a dark tan are not guarantees that you are getting sufficient vitamin D, especially as you age, since the capacity to activate vitamin D in the skin from sun exposure is lost over the years, particularly beyond age 40.

Avoid the D_2, or ergocalciferol, form, as it is nonhuman and not as effective or safe as the human form, D_3 or cholecalciferol. (D_2 is the form present in prescription vitamin D, but just because it's the prescription form does *not* make it better.) Because there is wide individual variation in vitamin D dose required to achieve the same target levels in the body, it helps to obtain an occasional blood test for 25-hydroxy vitamin D that reflects your vitamin D status. Ideally, blood levels should be assessed no sooner than 3 months after initiating supplementation (since it takes that long to plateau), then reassessed yearly to ensure that you remain within the target range.

Just as cultivation of bowel flora synergizes with the benefits of wheat and grain elimination, adding vitamin D to the mix adds yet another level of positive synergistic interaction that takes you even further down the path of restored health.

CORRECT MAGNESIUM DEFICIENCY

400 to 500 milligrams (mg) per day elemental magnesium as magnesium malate, glycinate, or chelate, divided into two or three doses

Recall that the phytates of wheat and grains block absorption of nutrients, mostly minerals. Magnesium is among those blocked, with absorption reduced by 60 percent in the presence of grains. Magnesium deficiency is further compounded by reliance on home or municipal water filtration that removes all magnesium from drinking water, by the reduced magnesium content of modern crops, and by widespread use of drugs for acid reflux and ulcers that reduce magnesium absorption. Add it all up, and magnesium deficiency is the *rule* at the start of your program. Unless corrected, magnesium deficiency will continue and impair your full recovery following grain elimination. We therefore work to restore magnesium.

The Recommended Dietary Allowance, or RDA, of "elemental" magnesium, i.e., magnesium by itself, is 320 mg per day for adult females and 420 mg per day for adult males. Most of us take in far less, with much absorption previously blocked by grains. Deficiency is associated with osteoporosis, hypertension, higher blood sugars, muscle cramps, migraine headaches, and heart rhythm disorders. Magnesium deficiency can express itself to an exaggerated degree during the wheat/grain withdrawal process, experienced as leg cramps and disruption of sleep during the first few days, so everyone ideally begins magnesium supplementation on Day 1 of the Wheat Belly lifestyle.

We therefore add a magnesium supplement at the start and aim to obtain 400 to 500 mg per day of elemental magnesium. We've got to be choosy with magnesium supplements, however, as most are better laxatives than forms of absorbable magnesium. Look for magnesium malate, magnesium glycinate, or magnesium chelate, which are among the best absorbed. You can also find a simple recipe to make your own magnesium water, a source of the best absorbed form of magnesium, magnesium bicarbonate, in *Wheat Belly Total Health* and *Wheat Belly 10-Day Grain Detox*. Regardless of what form of magnesium you choose, divide your daily intake into two or three doses per day to minimize potential for loose stools.

It also helps to increase intake of magnesium-rich foods, such as pumpkin seeds, sesame seeds, and sunflower seeds; nuts such as almonds and pecans, as well as peanuts and (unsweetened) peanut butter; and lots of spinach and other green leafy vegetables.

FISH OIL: THE *ONLY* SAFE AND ASSURED SOURCE OF OMEGA-3 FATTY ACIDS

3,000 to 3,600 mg per day of EPA + DHA from fish oil *only,* divided in two doses

Infrequent consumption of seafood, aversion to organ meats, and overreliance on processed omega-6 oils in modern foods have led to deficient levels of omega-3 fatty acids in the majority of people at the start of their program. Grains compound the problem with their absorption-blocking and inflammatory effects. Once grains are removed, omega-3 fatty acid absorption may improve, but intake typically remains low for most people so supplementation is necessary to achieve healthy blood levels.

There are plenty of other reasons to supplement omega-3 fatty acids. Clinical studies demonstrate that omega-3 fatty acids, as eicosapentaenoic acid (EPA) and docosahexaenoic acid (DHA) obtained from fish and fish oil, yield reductions in sudden cardiac death, heart attack, heart rhythm disorders, autoimmune inflammatory conditions (especially rheumatoid arthritis and lupus), and a variety of cancers. These potential benefits apply *only* to the EPA and DHA from fish and fish oil, not to the linolenic acid of flaxseeds, chia seeds, walnuts, and other sources. (While linolenic acid is biochemically an omega-3 fatty acid and is, for other reasons, a truly healthy oil, it does not yield the same benefits provided by EPA and DHA from fish.) Krill oil is likewise *not* a useful source of EPA and DHA for us, as the quantities contained are too small to achieve the benefits we desire (despite the over-the-top misleading marketing claims made by some manufacturers).

I advocate an intake of 3,000 to 3,600 mg per day of the EPA and DHA contained in fish oil (the dose of combined omega-3 fatty acids, EPA and DHA, not of the entire fish oil capsule that contains omega-3s and other oils), divided into two doses: one dose taken before breakfast, and another before or after dinner. This quantity yields an ideal level of omega-3 fatty acids in the bloodstream, subdues the flood of fatty acids after meals and during weight loss, provides maximal protection from cardiovascular disease, and yields anti-inflammatory benefits.

Fish oil by itself provides only modest benefits. But taken on the background of the combined Wheat Belly strategies of wheat/grain elimination, cultivation of healthy bowel flora, vitamin D restoration, etc., the benefits of fish oil further compound the benefits of this program, once again providing a powerful synergistic effect among the combined strategies.

IODINE: FORGOTTEN BUT VITAL NUTRIENT

500 to 1,000 micrograms (mcg) per day as kelp tablets or iodine drops (potassium iodide)

Iodine deficiency is making a big comeback with broad implications for health. Failure to correct iodine deficiency can substantially impair your ability to lose weight, while adding to cardiovascular risk, hypertension, water retention, fatigue, and risk for breast cancer.

Iodine is an essential trace mineral. Because salivary glands and breast tissue concentrate iodine, it is required for oral health and protection from conditions such as fibrocystic breast disease. Iodine is essential for normal thyroid function, in particular, since thyroid hormones, T4 and T3, are composed of iodine (the "4" and "3" referring to the number of iodine molecules). Iodine deficiency over time leads to a thyroid gland that enlarges—a goiter, seen as a bulge on the front of the neck. However, it is not necessary to have a goiter for thyroid dysfunction to be present.

The connection between goiter and iodine deficiency led to the introduction of iodized salt in 1924, and the FDA urged the public to use more salt. Unfortunately, excessive salt consumption caused health problems in some susceptible individuals, prompting new advice: Reduce salt and sodium consumption. Now, in the 21st century, health-conscious people avoid iodized table salt. Others have turned to alternative sources, such as sea salt (very little iodine content), kosher salt (no iodine), and potassium chloride–based salt substitutes (no iodine). Iodine content of iodized salt is inconsistent, evaporating from the container within 4 weeks of opening. This means that a canister of iodized salt that's been sitting, opened, in your cupboard for, say, 6 months contains little to no iodine. All of this leads to the reemergence of iodine deficiency, even goiters. While strategies such as wheat/grain elimination and cultivation of bowel flora are powerful tools for health, they will not restore iodine status. You specifically need to address iodine to correct deficiency.

Simply meeting the RDA of 150 mcg per day of iodine will prevent a goiter from developing but may not represent the ideal intake. Athletes and people engaged in frequent heavy physical effort have greater needs than the RDA because of iodine loss through perspiration. Vegetarians who avoid seafood and iodized salt also have a greater likelihood of iodine deficiency than omnivores. The needs of both groups may exceed the RDA.

I therefore advocate a daily iodine intake of 500 to 1,000 mcg (*not* milligrams), readily obtained from supplements such as potassium iodide drops or kelp tablets, dried seaweed that approximates the natural, ocean-derived source. (I prefer kelp, as it provides a mixture of iodine forms.)

TAKE ADVANTAGE OF THE
WHEAT BELLY 2 + 2 = 11 EFFECT

Put all the strategies of the Wheat Belly lifestyle to work and something very curious happens: Powerful synergies develop among each and every strategy. It also means that, leave out just one component, such as magnesium restoration or iodine supplementation, and you will dramatically impair the effectiveness of your program. I call this the Wheat Belly 2 + 2 = 11 effect in which the total is greater than the sum of the parts—*far* greater.

For example, people with type 2 diabetes who take the first Wheat Belly step of eliminating all wheat and grains and then tightly manage net carb intake (no more than 15 g net carbs per day) will drop blood sugars immediately and dramatically—but may not become nondiabetic right off. Add vitamin D and blood sugars, as well as blood pressure and triglycerides, drop further. Add magnesium and blood sugar fluctuations are subdued. Add efforts to cultivate healthy bowel flora and the body's responsiveness to insulin is markedly improved, further reducing blood sugar, blood pressure, and triglycerides. The combined effect stacks the odds in favor of someone making a full recovery from type 2 diabetes. Many other health conditions can also reap the full benefits of the Wheat Belly lifestyle when the same formula is adopted.

So resist the impulse to cherry-pick the strategies in the Wheat Belly lifestyle, and embrace each and every one to enjoy the full range of benefits and powerful synergies that emerge.

CHAPTER 5

WHEAT BELLY SAFE SWEETENERS

WE AVOID SWEETENERS with unhealthy consequences. We therefore banish sucrose (table sugar); fructose-containing sweeteners such as corn syrup, high-fructose corn syrup, and agave; and minimize honey and maple syrup as well as raw sugar, coconut nectar, coconut sugar, and other sugar products meant to conceal the fact that they are still sugar.

We obtain sweetness to re-create cookies, muffins, and other goodies by using safe, *natural* sweeteners that have little to no health downside, including no effect on your carb intake. In other words, these sweeteners, when used in the quantities specified in Wheat Belly recipes, will not interfere with blood sugar or weight loss or have other adverse consequences.

Our choices of safe sweeteners are:

- **ERYTHRITOL**—A natural sweetener naturally found in fruit, erythritol has 70 percent of the sweetness of sugar and minimal potential to raise blood sugar. It therefore takes a bit more than a 1:1 replacement with sugar to yield the same sweetness. For example, 4 teaspoons of erythritol provides the same sweetness as 3 teaspoons of sugar.

- **INULIN**—Inulin is obtained from root plants such as the Jerusalem artichoke, dandelion root, and chicory root. With only mild sweetness, inulin is best used in combination with other natural sweeteners. Inulin also acts as a prebiotic fiber to nourish bowel flora.
- **MONK FRUIT (ALSO KNOWN AS *LO HAN GUO*)**—This is another natural sweetener without calories, available as a liquid or nectar.
- **STEVIA**—Stevia is a natural sweetener from the leaf of the stevia plant. Look for pure liquid or pure powdered stevia. Avoid those bulked up with maltodextrin, which is essentially sugar. Highly concentrated and therefore pricey, stevia is surprisingly among the least expensive sweeteners, since a little goes a long way.
- **XYLITOL**—Another natural sweetener found in fruit, xylitol also has minimal capacity to raise blood sugar. (Be aware, however, that xylitol is toxic to dogs.) Pure xylitol can be used 1:1 in place of sugar: 1 tablespoon of xylitol yields the same sweetening power as 1 tablespoon of sucrose.

For stevia and monk fruit, there are no standard sweetening equivalents to sugar, as different brands can differ widely in concentration. The key is to stick to a brand you like and get comfortable with that brand's sweetening power. It is always advisable to taste your batter or other recipe-in-progress and adjust the sweetener.

Premixed combinations of sweeteners are also available, especially useful if you experience unpleasant aftertastes with stevia or erythritol alone. Unlike plain stevia or monk fruit, premixed combinations can replace sugar in predictable proportions. Wheat-Free Market Virtue Sweetener (erythritol and monk fruit) is four times sweeter than sugar: ¼ cup yields the sweetness of 1 cup of sugar. Lakanto (erythritol and monk fruit) and Swerve (inulin and erythritol) replace sugar 1:1. Truvia (erythritol and rebiana, an isolate of stevia) has twice the sweetness of sugar: ½ cup yields the sweetness of 1 cup of sugar.

If combinations of sweeteners and/or premixed combinations still yield an unpleasant aftertaste, another method is to use a small quantity of sugar, such as that provided by a handful of raisins, dates, or other natural sources combined with your sweetener(s) of choice from our list. For example, pulverize two medjool dates in your food chopper or food processor, then use half the usual quantity of stevia or erythritol. You may have to go through a bit of trial and error to find the combination that's sweet enough for your palate without the aftertaste. Also, remain aware of your net carb intake for any recipe you modify.

CHAPTER 6

SAFE FLOURS AND MEALS FOR WHEAT BELLY BAKING AND "BREADING"

DISMISSING ALL WHEAT and grains from your life means having to adapt to using new ingredients that allow you to re-create tasty and healthy pizza crusts, muffins, cookies, and other baked dishes. The meals and flours we choose should be healthy and not be responsible for causing health problems such as high blood sugars or inflammation, as grain-based flours do. Nor should they cause the awful health problems of common gluten-free replacement flours, such as cornstarch, tapioca starch, potato starch, and rice flour responsible for blood sugar and weight gain disasters. We just want healthy meals and flours so that a slice of pizza or cake can be enjoyed without health concerns and without sacrificing flavor.

There are a number of healthy replacement flours and meals that fit nicely into your Wheat Belly lifestyle. While single-source flours and meals can be used, best results are generally obtained by combining two or three different flours and meals, yielding a more cohesive, less crumbly, and tasty end result. For example, a common useful combination is 3½ cups almond meal, ¼ cup ground golden flaxseeds, and 2 tablespoons coconut flour.

I cannot stress this enough: Nobody should be using the gluten-free baking mixes or flours/meals made with the common gluten-free ingredients cornstarch, potato flour, rice flour, or tapioca starch. They send blood sugar sky-high and thereby provoke resistance to insulin, block weight loss and typically cause extravagant weight gain, and lead to the metabolic distortions that increase risk for diabetes, heart disease, cancer, and dementia. They can cause problems even if consumed occasionally, in "moderation"—yes, they are that bad. I urge you to never rely on such products, inconvenient or not, especially since we have safe and healthy alternative flours and meals that cause none of these problems.

For convenience and as a time-saver, I've included our All-Purpose Baking Mix recipe on page 51, a combination of meals, seeds, and flours that can be used to make just about any healthy, grain-free baked product.

Here's my list of safe meals and flours:

ALMOND FLOUR—Almond flour is ground from blanched almonds with the skins removed that may or may not have had excess oil pressed from it. This yields a finer flour than almond meal but minus much of the fiber. It is also more costly than the meal. I reserve the use of almond flour for situations in which a lighter texture is required, such as a layer cake or cupcakes.

ALMOND MEAL–This is the meal ground from whole almonds with the skin left on. It yields a coarser baked end product than almond flour but is typically less expensive. Shop around, as prices vary widely.

CHIA SEED MEAL–Much like ground flaxseeds (see below), this is best used as a secondary flour.

COCONUT FLOUR–The flour ground from coconut meat has a wonderful taste and scent (not coconut-y, for those of you who do not like coconut). However, it yields an exceptionally dense end product. I therefore only use coconut flour as a secondary flour to modify the taste and texture of a primary flour, such as almond meal. If a dense texture is desired, you can increase the proportion of coconut flour. However, be aware that using too much will yield a very dry end product. A typical combination would be 3½ cups of almond flour with 1 to 2 tablespoons of coconut flour.

GARBANZO BEAN FLOUR–Garbanzo beans have among the lowest carbohydrate content of the various bean flours available. But because garbanzo bean flour can still yield excessive carbs, I find it useful as a secondary flour, added for improved structure and cohesiveness.

GROUND GOLDEN FLAXSEEDS–It's the *golden* flaxseeds you want, not the more common brown, when you desire a flour replacement. The golden yields a finer texture with less of an "off" flavor. Used by itself, ground golden flaxseeds tend to be too crumbly, so it is best used as a secondary flour along with almond meal or other nut or seed meal.

GROUND PECANS—Pecans yield a coarser flour than that from almonds, but it can still be used in place of almond meal or flour. I find that ground pecans are perfect for creating pie crusts.

GROUND WALNUTS—Ground walnuts are coarser and best used as pie crust or in recipes in which a coarse texture is desired.

PUMPKIN SEED MEAL—Easy to grind, pumpkin seed meal yields a dense and useful all-around baking meal.

SESAME SEED MEAL—Sesame seeds yield a surprisingly light flour. Buy sesame seeds in bulk, which is far less expensive than the small jars in the spice aisle.

SUNFLOWER SEED MEAL—Like pumpkin seed meal, sunflower seed meal is a useful all-around meal. Avoid using baking soda or baking powder when using sunflower meal, as it will turn your baked products green (from chlorophyll). Should you use baking powder/soda and obtain a green, say, muffin, it is still perfectly safe to eat; it just looks funny.

CHAPTER 7

SAFE WHEAT BELLY THICKENERS FOR GRAVIES AND SAUCES

IN THE WHEAT BELLY lifestyle, we've removed all wheat flour and cornstarch commonly used to thicken gravies and sauces. Can you still have a tasty but healthy gravy with your Thanksgiving turkey or an appealing sauce with meats, poultry, or fish without booby-trapping health? Are there safe choices that, unlike standard ingredients, don't have adverse, sometimes devastating, health consequences?

Yes, indeed! There are a number of excellent choices, ingredients that can reliably thicken gravies and sauces with none of the health issues raised by wheat or corn products. I know of *no* dishes that cannot be accompanied by a gravy or sauce made from our rich choices of healthy alternative ingredients.

Because we don't want to replace one problem ingredient with another, like replacing unfiltered cigarettes with low-tar cigarettes, we choose benign, healthy thickening agents. For this reason, we avoid, for example, arrowroot; though not a grain, it is virtually pure carbohydrate that converts immediately to blood sugar. (Very small quantities, such as 1 teaspoon, can be safe, but you can quickly lose control over blood sugar issues when using more.) Our choice of safe thickeners is therefore free of concerns over blood sugar, inflammation, or weight gain.

Here are my top choices:

AVOCADO—Avocado (pureed in your food processor or food chopper) is a marvelous thickening agent for smoothies and puddings.

BUTTER—In general, dairy does not figure prominently in the Wheat Belly lifestyle, as there are issues with hormone content, whey protein, casein, and lactose. But butter, especially if organic, is among the least problematic dairy products, since it is almost entirely fat. The Wheat Belly lifestyle does not involve any restrictions on fat, saturated fat, or calories, so go to town with butter and enjoy its rich flavors and ability to thicken.

CHIA SEEDS, GROUND GOLDEN FLAXSEEDS—These are best for thickening puddings, jams, and smoothies as they tend to yield a not-so-desirable gooey texture you may not like for gravy. They perform their thickening function best by heating. For example, if you're making a strawberry sauce or jam, first puree the strawberries in a blender, food chopper, or food processor. Add them to a saucepan, then stir in chia seeds or ground golden flaxseeds over low heat, adding enough to obtain the desired thickness.

COCONUT FLOUR AND/OR CANNED COCONUT MILK— Coconut flour by itself or combined with coconut milk can make a great roux or gravy. The key is to add coconut flour slowly and sparingly while heating at a low temperature, e.g., low simmer in a saucepan, stirring in 1 teaspoon every minute or so. Because coconut flour is highly hygroscopic, or water-absorbent, impatience can lead to a pan of concrete rather than a nicely thickened gravy. That is why we add this thickening ingredient slowly. You can keep any coconut flavors from showing through by adding more sea salt, ground pepper, onion powder, ground thyme, or other seasonings. The end product will be a bit more gritty than that made with cornstarch or wheat flour (because of protein), but the flavor will be wonderful, especially if drippings or home-made stocks are used. Coconut milk will yield a thinner, though equally delicious, end result, without the grittiness. When used with coconut milk, coconut flour creates greater thickness.

HEAVY CREAM—Not my first choice due to my reservations about dairy products that contain more than dairy fat (see "Butter"). But, for occasional use, it is a versatile and delicious thickener. You can also add egg yolk to create a liaison for added richness, just as you would in traditional French cooking.

MUSHROOMS—I learned from Wheat Belly readers that pureed mushrooms, such as portobello, make a terrific thickener, adding another dimension of flavor. One caveat: A powerful chopper or food processor will be needed to generate a smooth puree, else you will get a grainy consistency.

NUT BUTTERS—Aside from peanut butter in Thai dishes, I find nut butters most useful for thickening nonsavory dishes, such as smoothies. Nut butters are also useful ingredients to create icings to spread on cupcakes, cakes, and other baked goodies, sweetened with one or a combination of safe natural sweeteners from the list starting on page 39.

OKRA—Unlike other veggies, okra does not have to be pureed, but can be added to, say, gumbo as it cooks on the stove. Like zucchini, it is low in net carbs with 4 g per cup.

PUREED EGGPLANT, ZUCCHINI, BROCCOLI, PUMPKIN, SQUASH—Vegetables can be wonderful ingredients to use for thickening. Just be mindful of carbohydrate exposure with higher carb choices such as squash. These thickeners are especially compatible with soups. Zucchini is the easiest and safest choice for most dishes, both sweet and savory, with 3 grams (g) net carbs per cup. Start by using only the pulp without the skin and pureeing in a blender, food chopper, or food processor to the desired consistency.

CHAPTER 8

WHEAT BELLY BASIC RECIPES

HERE IS A collection of basic recipes that allow you to make healthy grain-free breads, as well as mayonnaise, ketchup, salad dressings, and jams—the staples of everyday life that can be tough, sometimes impossible, to purchase without the ingredients we are trying to avoid (added sugar, high-fructose corn syrup, and unhealthy oils). If you are looking for additional recipes for day-to-day staples, such as icings for cakes or barbecue and other sauces, many more can be found in *Wheat Belly 30-Minute (or Less!) Cookbook*.

ALL-PURPOSE BAKING MIX

This is the baking mix I shared with Wheat Belly readers that has stood the test of time, yielding breads, muffins, cupcakes, and other grain-free baked products. Having this premixed helps shave a few minutes off preparation time.

Makes 5 cups

> 4 cups almond meal/flour
> 1 cup ground golden flaxseeds
> ¼ cup coconut flour
> 3 teaspoons baking soda
> 1 teaspoon ground psyllium seed

In a large bowl, combine all ingredients and mix well. Store in an airtight container, preferably in the refrigerator, for up to 1 month.

BASIC MINI SANDWICH BREADS

We use a whoopie pie baking pan as the mold in this virtually foolproof way to make breads for mini sandwiches. Remember, the Wheat Belly lifestyle is more filling than a wheat grain-containing diet, meaning even mini sandwiches can be surprisingly filling.

Makes 8

1½ cups All-Purpose Baking Mix (page 51)
¾ teaspoon sea salt
4 tablespoons extra-virgin or avocado oil
1 egg
1½ tablespoons water + additional if needed

Preheat the oven to 350°F. Lightly grease 8 cups of a whoopie pie baking pan.

In a medium bowl, combine the baking mix, salt, oil, egg, and water and mix thoroughly. Dough should be the consistency of thick pancake batter. If too thick, add more water, ½ tablespoon at a time. Divide the dough among the 8 cups of the baking pan, spread, and flatten.

Bake for 18 minutes, or until the edges just begin to brown. Remove from the oven and allow to cool before removing from the pan.

BASIC FOCACCIA

Generating "rise" in breads without grains is a perennial challenge. One solution is to make flatbreads, or focaccia, that can be every bit as tasty and versatile, though heavier in texture than conventional grain-based breads. You can liven up this basic focaccia recipe by adding sliced kalamata olives, tapenades, sun-dried tomatoes, or other herbs and spices.

Makes 15 slices

6 cups All-Purpose Baking Mix (page 51) or almond meal/flour
¼ cup ground psyllium seed (omit if using Baking Mix)
2 teaspoons ground rosemary
2 teaspoons dried oregano
2 teaspoons dried onion powder
2 teaspoons sea salt
5 eggs, separated
1 cup warm water
½ cup extra-virgin olive, avocado, or coconut oil or butter

Preheat the oven to 375°F. Grease an 11" x 17" shallow baking pan.

In a large bowl, combine the baking mix or almond meal/flour, psyllium seed (if using), rosemary, oregano, onion powder, and salt and stir until well blended.

In a medium bowl, combine the egg yolks, water, and oil or butter and whisk to combine.

In a large bowl and using an electric mixer on high, whip the egg whites until frothy and stiff.

Pour the egg yolk mixture and whipped egg whites into the flour mixture and combine thoroughly to create a dough. Transfer it to the baking pan and spread with a spoon or by hand to fill the pan edge to edge.

Bake for 18 minutes. Remove and cut the bread, using a knife or pizza cutter, lengthwise into 3 lengths and horizontally into 5, to yield 15 slices. Or cut into the sizes you desire.

MAYONNAISE

Store-bought mayonnaises are made with unhealthy oils, such as soybean and safflower oil. Making mayonnaise yourself can sometimes be tricky, but here is an easy version made with an immersion blender. The same process can be followed with a blender or food processor.

All ingredients must be at room temperature. If the ingredients are refrigerated, wait at least 2 hours to allow them to warm to room temperature before using, or else they will not blend properly.

Makes about 1½ cups

2 egg yolks
2 tablespoons white wine vinegar
1 cup extra-light olive or avocado oil
½ teaspoon salt

In a tall, narrow jar that accommodates an immersion blender, blend the egg yolks and vinegar for 15 to 20 seconds, or until frothy.

Pour in ¼ to ⅓ cup of the oil *very* slowly, over 2 to 3 minutes. As the mixture thickens, pour in the rest of the oil over 1 to 2 minutes while continuing to blend. Once it's thickened, add the salt.

Cover and store. The mayonnaise will keep in the refrigerator for up to 1 week.

KETCHUP

The problem with conventional store-bought ketchup is the high-fructose corn syrup or excessive sugars. Here is an easy way to make ketchup without added sweeteners.

Makes about 1 cup

1 can (6 ounces) tomato paste
¼ cup apple cider or white wine vinegar
¼ cup water
1½ teaspoons onion powder
1 teaspoon garlic powder
¼ teaspoon sea salt

In a small saucepan, combine the tomato paste, vinegar, water, onion powder, garlic powder, and salt. Cook over low heat, stirring occasionally, for 20 minutes.

Cool and store in an airtight container in the refrigerator for up to 2 weeks.

STRAWBERRY JAM

Here is a basic method to convert fruit to a spreadable jam using chia seeds. While this recipe calls for strawberries, it can be readily modified to use apricots, plums, or other berries or fruit.

Makes 2 cups

2 cups fresh strawberries
¼ cup whole chia seeds
Sweetener equivalent to ¾ cup sugar
1 tablespoon fresh-squeezed lemon juice

In a food processor or food chopper, pulse the strawberries until pureed.

Transfer to a small saucepan over low heat and stir in the chia seeds and sweetener. Stir frequently for 5 minutes, or until the mixture thickens.

Remove and allow to cool. Stir in the lemon juice when cooled. Store in the refrigerator, covered, for up to 1 week.

SALAD DRESSINGS

If you've become accustomed to store-bought salad dressings, then you are in for a treat. These are the real thing, with fresh and delightful flavors and none of the health problems.

SPICY CURRY DRESSING

This is a two-birds-with-one-stone salad dressing: Not only is it delicious and healthy, but it also provides prebiotic fibers for cultivation of healthy bowel flora by including hummus, a source of prebiotic fibers.

The exotic combination of flavors in garam masala—cinnamon, nutmeg, cloves, cardamom, and cumin—blend with those of red curry to make a delicious salad dressing or sauce for meats and other dishes. This dressing is best prepared and consumed on the same day you make it, as the spices of the garam masala tend to lose their flavors within several hours.

If used as a sauce on a hot dish, such as baked chicken or fish, add it during the last few moments of cooking to avoid excessive heating, which can degrade the prebiotic fibers into sugar.

Makes about 1½ cups

½ cup hummus
½ cup extra-virgin olive oil
¼ cup red curry paste
2 tablespoons apple cider vinegar
2 tablespoons water
1 teaspoon garam masala
1 teaspoon red-pepper flakes

In a small bowl, combine the hummus, oil, curry paste, vinegar, water, garam masala, and pepper flakes and mix thoroughly. Store in an airtight container in the refrigerator for no longer than 2 weeks.

ITALIAN TOMATO BASIL VINAIGRETTE

You can be confident that this vinaigrette contains no grains or added sugar, but it loses nothing in flavor.

Makes about 2½ cups

½ cup sun-dried tomatoes (oil-infused)
½ cup coarsely chopped fresh basil
2 cloves garlic, minced
1 cup extra-virgin olive oil
¼ tomato paste or ½ cup tomato sauce
½ cup apple cider, white wine, or red wine vinegar
½ teaspoon salt or to taste

Place the tomatoes, basil, garlic, oil, tomato paste or sauce, vinegar, and salt in a food processor or food chopper. Pulse until pureed.

Store in an airtight container in the refrigerator for up to 1 week.

FRENCH DRESSING

If you have made our Mayonnaise (page 54) and Ketchup (page 55), then this French Dressing is just a handful of additional ingredients away.

Makes about 2 cups

½ cup extra-virgin olive or avocado oil
½ cup Mayonnaise (page 54)
½ cup Ketchup (page 55)
⅓ cup white wine or apple cider vinegar
1 small onion, chopped
Sweetener equivalent to ¼ cup sugar
1 teaspoon paprika
½ teaspoon sea salt

In a blender, combine the oil, mayonnaise, ketchup, vinegar, onion, sweetener, paprika, and salt. Blend until well mixed.

Store in an airtight container in the refrigerator for up to 1 week.

CHAPTER 9

THE TOP 10 WHEAT BELLY RECIPES

HERE ARE THE recipes that, time and again, Wheat Belly readers make and proudly post their photos on social media, such as the Wheat Belly Facebook page. Most of these recipes have become so popular because they suit the tastes and needs of family members and friends—often surprising others when they realize just how delicious and rich this lifestyle can be. Please feel free to do likewise and post your photos!

CHICAGO-STYLE DEEP-DISH PEPPERONI PIZZA

Here's a real winner in the Wheat Belly lifestyle, a thick, luscious Chicago-style pizza that is virtually guaranteed to wow the family.

Even more than with conventional pizza crusts, it is important to use a thick pizza sauce to minimize the risk of a soggy crust. The sauce should be thick and not watery. If it's too thin, simmer over low heat for at least 30 minutes, stirring occasionally, to remove the excess moisture.

I specify a cast-iron or ovenproof skillet in this recipe, but a deep-dish pizza pan works well, too.

Makes 4 servings

8 tablespoons extra-virgin olive oil, divided
2 cups almond meal/flour or All-Purpose Baking Mix (page 51)
½ teaspoon sea salt
1 tablespoon chopped fresh basil or 1 teaspoon dried
2 tablespoons chopped fresh oregano or 2 teaspoons dried
1 cup shredded mozzarella cheese, divided
2 large eggs
¼ cup water
1 small onion, minced
1 small bell pepper, chopped
1 jar (14 ounces) pizza sauce
4 ounces pepperoni, sliced

Preheat the oven to 375°F. Grease the bottom and sides of a large cast-iron skillet (10" diameter) or other ovenproof skillet with 1 tablespoon of the oil.

In a medium bowl, combine the almond meal/flour or baking mix, salt, basil, oregano, and ½ cup of the cheese. In a small bowl, whisk together the eggs and 2 tablespoons of the oil, then stir in the water. Pour the egg mixture into the almond mixture and mix thoroughly. Set aside.

Place the onion, pepper, and 1 tablespoon of the oil in the prepared skillet over medium-high heat and cook for 3 minutes, or until the onion is translucent. Remove from the heat and transfer the onion mixture to a bowl. Pour off any liquid from the bowl.

Allow the skillet to cool for several minutes. Then, using a spatula or large spoon, press the dough evenly into the pan, tracking up the sides at least 1". Bake for 15 minutes and remove from oven. (Hot! Use an oven mitt.)

Top with the pizza sauce, onion mixture, pepperoni, and the remaining ½ cup cheese, and drizzle with the remaining 4 tablespoons of oil. Bake for 10 minutes, or until the cheese is melted.

"SPAGHETTI" WITH MEATBALLS

This recipe includes spiral-cut zucchini, or what some call "zoodles." You will need one of the low-cost spiral-cutting devices, such as a Spirelli, Spiralizer, or one of the many others now on the market. While you could make do with a knife or mandolin, the spiral cutters are so much easier and quicker to use, and they generate thinner, more noodle-like slices— well worth the modest investment.

If you choose to use a store-bought tomato sauce, be sure to choose a brand with the least sugar and, whenever possible, choose brands (such as Muir Glen) that use BPA-free cans for tomatoes and tomato paste. Alternatively, make your own sauce from the recipe below, but be sure and do that first since it cooks for quite a while.

Makes 4 servings

"SPAGHETTI" AND MEATBALLS

1½ pounds ground beef
¼ cup ground golden flaxseeds
1 egg
1 tablespoon chopped fresh basil or 1 teaspoon dried
1 tablespoon chopped fresh oregano or 1 teaspoon dried
1 teaspoon sea salt
1 tablespoon extra-virgin olive oil
1 medium onion, chopped
3 or 4 cloves garlic, minced
1½ pounds zucchini, spiral cut
1 jar (28 ounces) store-bought tomato sauce, or homemade
     tomato sauce (recipe follows)

HOMEMADE TOMATO SAUCE

1 small onion, chopped
3 cloves garlic, minced
4 tablespoons extra-virgin olive oil, divided

2 cans (28 ounces each) whole peeled tomatoes
1 can (6 ounces) tomato paste
1 teaspoon sea salt + extra to taste
1 tablespoon chopped fresh basil or 1 teaspoon dried
1 tablespoon chopped fresh oregano or 1 teaspoon dried
Ground black pepper to taste

To make the "spaghetti" and meatballs: In a medium bowl, combine the beef, flaxseeds, egg, basil, oregano, and salt and mix by hand until thoroughly combined. Form into 1" balls.

In a large skillet over medium-high heat, add the oil, onion, and garlic and cook for 3 minutes, or until the onion is translucent. Add the meatballs and cook, turning occasionally, for 10 minutes, or until lightly browned on all surfaces and cooked through. Using a slotted spoon, transfer the meatballs and onion mixture to a large bowl and cover.

Add the zucchini to the skillet, cover, and cook, tossing occasionally, for 3 minutes, or until softened but not limp.

To make the sauce: In a large skillet, cook the onion and garlic in 1 tablespoon of the oil over medium-high heat for 3 minutes, or until the onion is translucent.

Meanwhile, pour the tomatoes into a blender and blend briefly until reduced to puree.

Transfer the tomatoes to the onion-garlic mixture, followed by the tomato paste, salt, and the remaining 3 tablespoons oil. Cover, reduce the heat to low, and simmer for 1½ hours. Stir in the basil, oregano, pepper, and additional salt to taste, then serve.

Serve the noodles topped with the meatballs and the tomato sauce.

PEANUT BUTTER COOKIES

Use the perennial favorite, peanut butter, to win the entire family over to the grain-free side of healthy eating.

For an extra-special treat, dip one-half of each cookie into melted 85% cocoa chocolate and cool on waxed or parchment paper.

While we avoid sugar-containing sweeteners in general, using small quantities distributed throughout a recipe can be safe. Here I use a touch of molasses for cohesiveness and color and to illustrate a way to reduce reliance on other sweeteners, especially if you are among those who experience a bitter aftertaste with stevia.

Makes 20

1 cup almond meal/flour
½ cup finely chopped walnuts
1 teaspoon ground cinnamon
Sweetener equivalent to ¾ cup sugar
2 eggs
2 cups peanut butter, at room temperature
1 stick (4 ounces) butter, melted, or ½ cup coconut oil, melted
1 tablespoon molasses
1 teaspoon vanilla extract

Preheat the oven to 350°F. Line a shallow baking sheet with parchment paper.

In a large bowl, stir together the almond meal/flour, walnuts, cinnamon, and sweetener.

In a medium-size bowl, whisk the eggs, then stir in the peanut butter, butter or coconut oil, molasses, and vanilla. Mix thoroughly, then pour into the bowl with the dry ingredients and stir until combined.

Spoon the mixture into about 20 1½" to 2" diameter, ¾" high mounds, pressing and shaping with a large spoon. Bake for 15 minutes, or until very lightly browned.

BREAKFAST CHEESECAKE

Yes, cheesecake for breakfast! Made ahead of time, this simple and light cheesecake can be a special treat to start your morning. Because it is made with ricotta, rather than cream cheese, it is lighter in texture than standard cheesecake. And it's not just for breakfast; this recipe can serve as a light dessert, too.

Optionally, serve with nonsugary Strawberry Jam (page 56) or other non-sugar-containing jam or preserve, or simply berries.

Makes 8 servings

1 cup ricotta cheese, at room temperature
½ cup coconut flour
Sweetener equivalent to ¼ cup sugar
4 teaspoons lemon juice
4 eggs, separated
1 teaspoon vanilla extract

Preheat the oven to 375°F. Grease a 9" x 9" baking pan.

In a medium bowl, place the ricotta, flour, sweetener, lemon juice, egg yolks, and vanilla.

In another medium bowl, with an electric mixer on high speed, beat the egg whites until stiff peaks form. Using the same beaters, beat the ricotta mixture until smooth. With a spoon, gently fold the egg whites into the ricotta mixture until thoroughly combined.

Pour into the baking pan. Bake for 20 minutes, or until the edges begin to brown and a wooden pick inserted in the center comes out clean. Cool slightly before serving.

APRICOT GINGER GRANOLA

Here's your answer to breakfast cereal—but this "granola" has none of the problems of the products that line an entire aisle at your supermarket. Serve this granola mix with unsweetened coconut milk or almond milk, cold or hot.

This recipe uses a modest quantity of fruit sugar from apricots. If it's not sweet enough for, say, your 7-year-old, a few raisins sprinkled on top or a bit of stevia or your choice of sweetener can be added. Dried apricots allow you to minimize the use of the sweetener, while adding only around 20 grams (g) of net carbohydrates to the entire batch.

Use leftovers as a snack. This granola can be stored in an air-tight container at room temperature and will keep for about a week—longer if refrigerated.

Makes 10 cups

5 dried apricots
¼ cup coconut oil, melted
2 teaspoons vanilla extract
½ teaspoon almond extract
2 cups raw sunflower seeds
2 cups raw pumpkin seeds
1 cup raw chopped pecans
1 cup raw sliced almonds
3 cups unsweetened shredded coconut or coconut flakes
1 teaspoon ground ginger
1 teaspoon allspice
Sweetener equivalent to ¼ cup sugar (optional)

Preheat the oven to 275°F.

In a food processor or food chopper, pulse the apricots until they are reduced to very small fragments. Transfer to a small bowl, add the oil, and mix thoroughly. Mix in the vanilla and almond extracts. Set aside.

In a large bowl, place the sunflower seeds, pumpkin seeds, pecans, almonds, coconut, ginger, allspice, and sweetener (if using) and mix. Stir in the apricot mixture until well mixed.

Spread the mixture in a large baking pan and bake for 7 to 8 minutes. Stir, then bake an additional 7 to 8 minutes, or until lightly browned. Remove and cool.

CREAM OF BROCCOLI SOUP

With the use of a blender, this wonderfully filling and simple variation on cream of broccoli soup can be whipped up in just a few minutes. We use coconut milk (the thicker canned variety) to take advantage of its satiating properties, positive health effects, and great taste.

Makes 6 servings

¼ cup butter, coconut oil, or extra-virgin olive oil
1 medium yellow onion, coarsely chopped
2 cloves garlic, coarsely chopped
4 cups chicken stock
1 pound broccoli florets, fresh or frozen
1 can (14 ounces) coconut milk
Salt and pepper to taste

In a large pot over medium-high heat, add the butter or oil and cook the onion and garlic for 3 minutes, or until the onion is translucent. Increase the heat to high and add the chicken stock. Bring to a boil, then reduce the heat to medium. Add the broccoli, milk, salt, and pepper and cook, stirring occasionally, for 5 minutes, or until the broccoli has softened.

Pour the mixture into a blender and puree. Alternatively, use a handheld immersion blender.

MEDITERRANEAN "PASTA" SALAD

You will be able to create a delicious pasta salad for picnics, summer gatherings, and other occasions, as well as a dish to enjoy during your Detox, by using this grain-free version using spiral-cut zucchini (see page 62) for the noodles.

Shorter noodles work best in this dish. Spiral-cut the noodles with short strokes to create noodles that are no more than 1½" to 2" in length. The flavors in this "pasta" salad are highlighted by the herbs, so choose fresh herbs whenever possible.

Makes 8 servings

1 pound zucchini, spiral-cut with short strokes
8 ounces cherry tomatoes, halved
1 medium cucumber, quartered and sliced
5 or 6 green onions, finely sliced
½ cup black or kalamata olives, pitted, halved, or sliced
8 ounces pepperoni, quartered and sliced
2 tablespoons chopped fresh basil or 2 teaspoons dried
1 tablespoon chopped fresh oregano or 1 teaspoon dried
¼ cup white vinegar
¼ cup extra-virgin olive oil
¼ cup grated Parmesan or Romano cheese (optional)

In a large bowl, combine the zucchini, tomatoes, cucumber, onions, olives, pepperoni, basil, oregano, vinegar, and oil and toss until well mixed. Top with the cheese, if using.

EGGPLANT LASAGNA

Rich and satisfying, this lasagna will make you forget you ever made the recipe using grains.

As a time-saver, use bottled marinara sauce, but choose brands with the least or no sugar added and certainly no high-fructose corn syrup. Nowadays, you can find many brands with no more than 10 to 12 g net carbs (total carbs—fiber) per 8 ounces of sauce on most store shelves.

Makes 8 servings

2 medium eggplants
2 tablespoons sea salt
1 cup extra-virgin olive oil, divided
1 jar (24 ounces) marinara sauce
2 tablespoons chopped fresh basil or 2 teaspoons dried
¼ cup chopped fresh oregano or 1 tablespoon dried
2 cups ricotta cheese
½ cup grated Parmesan cheese
1 large egg
2 cups shredded mozzarella cheese

Remove the ends of the eggplant, then cut lengthwise into ¼" slices. (Thinner pieces will brown more readily and yield more tender "noodles.") Cut the larger slices from the center in half to make narrower noodles. Place them in a colander over the sink and toss with the salt. Let sit for at least 30 minutes to allow the water to drain.

Rinse the eggplant briefly to remove the excess salt and drain. Working in batches, place the eggplant in a large skillet with 2 tablespoons of the oil over medium-high heat and cook for 2 to 3 minutes per side, or until brown. Add more oil with each batch as needed. Set aside.

In a medium saucepan, combine the marinara sauce, basil, and oregano and simmer over medium heat, stirring occasionally, for 15 to 20 minutes. Do not boil.

Preheat the oven to 375°F.

In a medium bowl, combine the ricotta, Parmesan, and egg and mix thoroughly.

Arrange one layer of eggplant on the bottom of a 9" x 13" baking dish. Top with the entire ricotta cheese mixture, then about 2 cups of the marinara sauce mixture. Layer the remaining eggplant, followed by the remaining marinara sauce. Top with the mozzarella.

Bake for 45 minutes, or until the cheese is lightly browned.

MASHED "POTATOES"

Although not a grain, potatoes yield too many carbohydrates when cooked. Excessive carbohydrates turn off your ability to lose weight by triggering blood sugar and insulin to high levels. Here is a way to not just replace mashed potatoes, but create something that tastes *even better*, with none of the health problems.

Replace butter with extra-virgin olive oil for a dairy-free version.

Makes 4 servings

1 large head cauliflower, cut into florets
¼ cup canned coconut milk
2 tablespoons butter
¼ teaspoon sea salt
Ground black pepper to taste

Place a steamer basket in a large pot with 2" water. Bring to a boil over high heat. Place the cauliflower in the basket, cover, and steam for 20 minutes, or until soft.

Remove from the heat and drain. In a blender, food processor, or food chopper, combine the cauliflower, coconut milk, butter, salt, and pepper. Blend or process until smooth.

"FETTUCCINE" ALFREDO

Rich and delicious, this can be served as a main dish or a substantial side dish.

Cheese and butter are among the most benign forms of dairy. Cheese is fermented, thereby reducing exposure to the casein protein. Butter is nearly all fat, avoiding exposure to the problematic dairy proteins. Because this is a dairy-rich dish, you can reduce the dairy, if desired, by replacing the cream with canned coconut milk and the butter with extra-virgin olive oil.

Serve with steamed green beans, broccoli, or other green vegetable or salad.

Makes 4 servings

½ cup grated Parmesan cheese
¾ cup grated Romano cheese
4 tablespoons butter
2 cloves garlic, minced
2 pounds zucchini, spiral-cut into fettuccine noodles
½ cup heavy cream or canned coconut milk
Sea salt and ground black pepper to taste

In a large bowl, mix together the Parmesan and Romano. Set aside.

In a large skillet over medium heat, melt the butter, add the garlic, and cook until it is just fragrant. Add the zucchini and cover, tossing occasionally, for 3 minutes, or until softened but not wilted. Add the cream or milk and bring to a light simmer. Add the salt and pepper, then remove from the heat.

Pour the mixture into the bowl with the cheeses, toss, and serve.

CHAPTER 10

A WHEAT BELLY 7-DAY MENU PLAN

HERE IS A sample 7-day menu plan drawing from the "basic" recipes in Chapter 8, the Top 10 Wheat Belly Recipes in Chapter 9, and selected recipes from *Wheat Belly Cookbook*, *Wheat Belly 30-Minute (or Less!) Cookbook*, and *Wheat Belly 10-Day Grain Detox*. Recipes from Chapter 9 are marked with an asterisk (*) along with the page number they appear on. Recipes excerpted from other *Wheat Belly* books are found in the section titled "Wheat Belly 7-Day Menu Plan Recipes" (page 77).

You will see that, in following the Wheat Belly lifestyle, you can take great liberties with your diet. You can have, for example, cheesecake for breakfast or make cookies an important part of lunch. You can do so because we re-create such familiar treats without wheat or grains and without added sugars, converting previously unhealthy foods into healthy replacements that can fit into any meal without impairing health. You also will likely find that three meals per day taken from recipes on the menu plan are incredibly filling, leaving you with plenty of leftovers. That's okay: Save leftovers for another meal, even if it means not following the meal plan precisely.

You can purchase all the necessary ingredients to create all the dishes on this menu plan by using "A Wheat Belly Shopping List to Follow the 7-Day Menu Plan" on page 96.

WHEAT BELLY 7-DAY MENU PLAN

DAY 1

BREAKFAST: Apricot Ginger Granola* (page 66) with unsweetened coconut/almond/hemp milk

LUNCH: Muffuletta Sandwiches (page 80)

DINNER: Mediterranean "Pasta" Salad* (page 69)

DAY 2

BREAKFAST: Jumbo Gingerbread Nut Muffins (page 78)

LUNCH: Thai Chicken Curry Soup (page 81)

DINNER: Chicago-Style Deep-Dish Pepperoni Pizza* (page 60)

DAY 3

BREAKFAST: Breakfast Cheesecake* (page 65)

LUNCH: BLT sandwich on Basic Focaccia (page 53)

DINNER: Roasted Brussels Sprouts and Ham Skillet (page 82)

DAY 4

BREAKFAST: Chorizo Frittata (page 83)

LUNCH: Grilled Cheese Sandwiches (opposte page)

DINNER: "Fettucine" Alfredo* (page 73)

DAY 5

BREAKFAST: Triple-Berry Quick Muffin (page 84)

LUNCH: Cream of Broccoli Soup* (page 68)

DINNER: Baked chicken, steamed broccoli or asparagus, with Mashed "Potatoes"* (page 72)

DAY 6

BREAKFAST: Mediterranean Scramble (page 85)

LUNCH: Spicy Minestrone (page 86) with Peanut Butter Cookies* (page 64)

DINNER: "Spaghetti" with Meatballs* (page 62)

DAY 7

BREAKFAST: Greek Frittata (page 87)

LUNCH: Egg salad sandwich or sloppy Joe on Basic Focaccia (page 53)

DINNER: Eggplant Lasagna* (page 70)

WHEAT BELLY 7-DAY MENU PLAN RECIPES

GRILLED CHEESE SANDWICHES

From *Wheat Belly Cookbook*

Nothing says comfort food like grilled cheese—until, of course, you suffer all the discomfort of having consumed something made of wheat! So here it is again, all comfort with no discomfort.

Try adding slices of tomato, red onion, fresh basil, or avocado for a change of pace. I like changing the cheese from the traditional Cheddar to Swiss or Gruyère for a slightly different spin.

Makes 4 servings

8 teaspoons butter
8 slices Basic Focaccia (page 53)
8 slices Cheddar cheese

Spread 1 teaspoon butter on each of 4 slices of bread. Place in a large nonstick skillet, buttered side down. Top each with 2 slices of cheese and a slice of bread. Spread each top slice with 1 teaspoon butter.

Cook over medium heat for 7 minutes, turning once, or until the bread is browned and the cheese is melted.

JUMBO GINGERBREAD NUT MUFFINS

From *Wheat Belly 10-Day Grain Detox*

They may not seem sufficient to stand alone as breakfast or lunch, but once you try these jumbo-size, nut- and oil-rich muffins, you will appreciate how filling they are. Because they are made with eggs, coconut oil, almonds, and other nuts and seeds, they are also very healthy. You can add a schmear of cream cheese or a bit of unsweetened fruit butter for added flavor. To fill out a lunch, add a chunk of cheese, some fresh berries or sliced fruit, or an avocado. While walnuts and pumpkin seeds are called for in the recipe to add crunch, you can substitute your choice of nut or seed, such as pecans, pistachios, or sunflower seeds.

As with any Wheat Belly recipe in which one of our benign sweeteners is used, adjust the quantity of sweetener to your tastes. Your perception of sweetness is sharpened the longer you are wheat- and grain-free, making you more and more sensitive to less and less sweetener.

A jumbo muffin tin is used in this recipe, but a smaller muffin tin can also be used. If a smaller tin is used, reduce the cooking time by about 5 minutes, though always assess by inserting a wooden pick into the center of a muffin and making sure that it withdraws clean. If you make the smaller size, pack two muffins for lunch.

Makes 6

4 cups almond meal/flour
1 cup shredded unsweetened coconut
½ cup chopped walnuts
½ cup pumpkin seeds
Sweetener equivalent to ¾ cup sugar
2 teaspoons ground cinnamon
1 tablespoon ground ginger
1 teaspoon ground nutmeg
½ teaspoon ground cloves
1 teaspoon sea salt

3 eggs
½ cup coconut oil, melted
1 teaspoon vanilla extract
½ cup water

Preheat the oven to 350°F. Place paper liners in a 6-cup jumbo muffin pan or grease the cups with coconut or other oil.

In a large bowl, combine the almond meal/flour, coconut, walnuts, pumpkin seeds, sweetener, cinnamon, ginger, nutmeg, cloves, and salt. Mix well.

In a medium bowl, whisk the eggs. Stir in the oil, vanilla, and water. Pour the egg mixture into the almond meal mixture and combine thoroughly.

Divide the batter evenly among the muffin cups. Bake for 30 minutes, or until a wooden pick inserted in the center of a muffin comes out clean.

MUFFULETTA SANDWICHES

From *Wheat Belly 30-Minute (or Less!) Cookbook*

This traditional New Orleans sandwich, dripping with olive oil and chopped olives, comes in many different versions, each with enthusiastic followers. Besides not using wheat-based bread, I depart from the usual routine by using Asiago cheese for an extra-cheesy "kick."

Muffuletta is properly served on sesame seed–coated bread. If adhering to tradition is important to you, make your Basic Focaccia with sesame seeds sprinkled on top.

Makes 4 servings

4 slices Basic Focaccia (page 53)
¼ cup muffuletta spread or tapenade
4 ounces sliced ham
2 ounces sliced pepperoni
2 ounces sliced mortadella
4 ounces sliced provolone cheese
2 ounces sliced Asiago cheese

Spread 2 slices of focaccia with the muffuletta spread or tapenade. Top evenly with the ham, pepperoni, mortadella, provolone, and Asiago. Top with the remaining 2 slices of focaccia. Carefully slice each sandwich in half.

THAI CHICKEN CURRY SOUP

From *Wheat Belly Cookbook*

With this flavorful variation on chicken soup, you will show your family that you can do anything a Thai restaurant can do. Serve this soup alongside a salad of fresh greens, watercress, and shredded carrots.

Makes 4 servings

2 tablespoons olive or coconut oil, divided

¾ pound boneless, skinless chicken thighs, cut into strips

3 ribs celery, sliced

3 cloves garlic, chopped

1 onion, chopped

1 red bell pepper, chopped

1 tablespoon minced fresh ginger

3 cups chicken broth

1 can (13.6 ounces) coconut milk

1 tablespoon green curry paste

2 tablespoons Thai fish sauce or gluten-free soy sauce

¼ cup chopped fresh cilantro

In a large pot over medium-high heat, heat 1 tablespoon of the oil. Cook the chicken, stirring, for 8 minutes, or until browned. Remove to a plate and keep warm.

In the same pot, heat the remaining 1 tablespoon oil. Cook the celery, garlic, onion, pepper, and ginger, stirring occasionally, for 3 minutes. Add the broth, coconut milk, curry paste, fish sauce or soy sauce, and the reserved chicken. Bring to a boil over high heat. Reduce the heat to low and simmer, stirring occasionally, for 4 minutes, or until the chicken is no longer pink and the vegetables are tender-crisp. Sprinkle with the cilantro.

ROASTED BRUSSELS SPROUTS AND HAM SKILLET

From *Wheat Belly 10-Day Grain Detox*

Here is another example of having breakfast for dinner. (The opposite concept—dinner for breakfast—works equally well in this lifestyle.) After all, we have turned the traditional notion of a grain-based breakfast inside out, breaking all the former "rules" of what is for breakfast and what is for dinner.

I snuck a sweet potato into this recipe for a bit of beta-carotene and flavor, adding only 5 grams net carbs per serving. The eggs are optional in this recipe, in case you don't want to take the breakfast-for-dinner idea all the way through.

Makes 4 servings

2 tablespoons extra-virgin olive oil or coconut oil
2 cloves garlic, minced
1 yellow onion, chopped
1 pound Brussels sprouts, halved
½ cup portobello mushrooms, sliced
1 medium sweet potato, chopped into ½-inch cubes
1 teaspoon sea salt
12 ounces precooked ham, cubed
4 eggs (optional)
¼ cup grated Parmesan cheese (optional)

Preheat the oven to 350°F.

In a large ovenproof skillet over medium-high heat, heat the oil. Cook the garlic and onion for 2 minutes, or until the onion is translucent. Add the Brussels sprouts, mushrooms, sweet potato, and salt and stir. Cook, covered, stirring occasionally, for 7 to 8 minutes, or until the Brussels sprouts and mushrooms soften. Stir in the ham.

If desired, use a spoon to form 4 small, evenly spaced depressions in the mixture. Crack an egg into each. Sprinkle the cheese over the top, if using.

Transfer the skillet to the oven and bake for 10 minutes.

CHORIZO FRITTATA

From *Wheat Belly 30-Minute (or Less!) Cookbook*

Using chorizo sausage in this frittata saves you the effort of adding spices and flavorings—because they're already in the sausage! Combine the spice of chorizo with the healthy green of kale and you have a perfect, healthy combination that is filling. Make the frittata ahead of time, refrigerate, and eat it over the course of the week for an entire week's worth of healthy breakfasts.

Makes 8 servings

2 tablespoons coconut oil
6 ounces chorizo sausage, chopped
1 yellow onion, chopped
2 cloves garlic, minced
1 cup fresh or frozen and thawed kale, chopped
½ cup sun-dried tomatoes, coarsely chopped
½ cup sliced baby bella mushrooms
10 eggs
½ teaspoon sea salt

Preheat the oven to 375°F.

In a large ovenproof skillet over medium-high heat, heat the oil. Cook the sausage, onion, and garlic for 3 minutes, or until the sausage is barely pink and the onion begins to soften. Reduce the heat to medium. Stir in the kale, tomatoes, and mushrooms. Cover and cook, stirring frequently, for 4 minutes, or until the mushrooms are tender.

Meanwhile, in a medium bowl, whisk the eggs and salt. Add to the skillet and gently tilt to distribute the eggs. Cook for 2 minutes, or until the bottom and edges of the egg mixture become slightly firm. Transfer to the oven and bake for 10 minutes, or until the center is nearly set.

TRIPLE-BERRY QUICK MUFFIN

From *Wheat Belly 30-Minute (or Less!) Cookbook*

These simple muffins require only about 3 minutes to make and are packed with healthy nuts (from the Baking Mix), berries, and plenty of protein and good-for-you fats. For crunch, consider adding dry-roasted (unsalted) pistachios or cashew, walnut, or pecan pieces.

Makes 1

½ cup All-Purpose Baking Mix (page 51)
¼ teaspoon ground cinnamon
Sweetener equivalent to 1 tablespoon sugar
Pinch of sea salt
1 egg
2 tablespoons whole milk, coconut or almond milk, or water
1 tablespoon butter or coconut oil, melted
¼ cup frozen or fresh mixed berries (blueberries, strawberries, blackberries)

In a medium bowl, combine the baking mix, cinnamon, sweetener, and salt. Whisk in the egg. Add the milk, butter, and berries and whisk thoroughly.

Use a rubber spatula to scrape the mixture into a large mug or a 10-ounce ramekin.

Microwave on high power for 2 minutes, or until a wooden pick inserted in the center comes out clean. (If using fresh berries, microwave for 1½ minutes.) Allow to cool for 5 minutes.

MEDITERRANEAN SCRAMBLE

From *Wheat Belly 30-Minute (or Less!) Cookbook*

To bring out the full, rich character of this healthy Mediterranean egg dish, use pasture-raised eggs whenever possible, the kind with orange-colored yolks that burst with flavor and contain higher nutrient content than mass-market eggs typically sold.

Makes 4 servings

4 tablespoons extra-virgin olive oil, divided
8 ounces Italian sausage, thinly sliced
1 small onion, finely chopped
2 cloves garlic, minced
1 can (14 ounces) quartered artichoke hearts, drained and
    chopped
¼ cup sun-dried tomatoes, finely chopped
¼ cup pitted kalamata olives, sliced
8 eggs
½ cup crumbled feta cheese

In a large skillet over medium heat, heat 2 tablespoons of the oil. Cook the sausage for 3 minutes, or until it starts to brown. Add the onion and garlic and cook, stirring occasionally, for 3 minutes, or until the onion is soft and the sausage is no longer pink.

Stir in the remaining 2 tablespoons oil, the artichokes, tomatoes, and olives.

In a medium bowl, whisk the eggs and pour into the skillet. Cook for 4 minutes, stirring occasionally, or until the eggs are set. Remove from the heat and gently stir in the cheese.

SPICY MINESTRONE

From *Wheat Belly 10-Day Grain Detox*

Don't you love how the flavors of vegetables mingle in a good minestrone? Here, we jazz it up a bit further with some peppery hot sauce and basil.

Makes 6 servings

4 tablespoons extra-virgin olive oil, divided
1 onion, chopped
2 cloves garlic, minced
4 cups chicken broth
4 cups water
1 can (14 ounces) diced tomatoes
1 can (6 ounces) tomato paste
2 teaspoons hot sauce
2 ribs celery, chopped
1 cup green beans, cut into 1" pieces
1 can (15 ounces) pinto beans
½ cup portobello or button mushrooms, sliced
1½ teaspoons sea salt + extra to taste
1 teaspoon ground black pepper + extra to taste
4 cups chopped fresh spinach or 1 box (10 ounces) frozen and
     thawed chopped spinach
¼ cup chopped fresh basil

In a large stockpot over medium-high heat, heat 1 tablespoon of the oil. Cook the onion and garlic, stirring frequently, for 2 to 3 minutes, or until softened.

Increase the heat to high and add the broth, water, tomatoes, tomato paste, hot sauce, celery, green beans, pinto beans, mushrooms, salt, pepper, and the remaining 3 tablespoons oil. Cover and bring to boil. Reduce the heat and simmer, partially covered, for 15 minutes.

Add the spinach and basil and cook for 10 minutes, or until the vegetables are tender. Taste and adjust the salt and pepper, if needed.

GREEK FRITTATA

From *Wheat Belly Cookbook*

In this modern collision of Greek and Italian, the rich tastes of kalamata olives, artichokes, sun-dried tomatoes, and fresh basil come together for a simple-to-prepare dish perfect for breakfast, lunch, dinner, or brunch. For convenience, prepare it on the weekend and store in the refrigerator to eat during the week.

Makes 6 servings

8 eggs

2 tablespoons half-and-half, heavy cream, or coconut milk
(canned)

1 tablespoon extra-virgin olive oil

½ red onion, chopped

¼ cup pitted kalamata olives, chopped

½ cup artichoke hearts, finely chopped

¼ cup sun-dried tomatoes (soaked in oil), chopped

2 tablespoons chopped fresh basil

½ cup finely crumbled feta cheese

½ teaspoon ground black pepper

Preheat the oven to 350°F.

In a medium bowl, whisk the eggs and half-and-half, cream, or coconut milk. Set aside.

In an ovenproof skillet over medium heat, heat the oil. Cook the onion, stirring frequently, for 5 minutes or until softened. Add the olives, artichokes, tomatoes, basil, cheese, and pepper. Cook for 5 minutes, or until the onion is browned.

Stir in the egg mixture. Cook for 3 minutes. Place in the oven and bake for 15 minutes, or until a knife inserted in the center comes out clean.

Using a spatula, release the frittata around the edges and bottom, and slide it onto a cutting board. Cool for 5 minutes, then cut into 6 wedges.

CHAPTER 11

WHEAT BELLY SHOPPING LISTS

HERE IS A list of many of the ingredients you will need to confidently follow a healthy Wheat Belly grain-free lifestyle. The items on this list are obviously going to differ from many of the foods, especially processed products, that you may already be familiar with, but there will be some overlap. We will also bring back some foods that you may have excluded from your diet because you were persuaded by conventional dietary advice that they were unhealthy—foods that would make your grandmother smile.

For simplicity, I won't list obviously healthy foods that probably already have a place in your kitchen, such as spinach, asparagus, mushrooms, fresh garlic, extra-virgin olive oil, organic butter, and eggs, as well as common herbs and spices such as cinnamon and nutmeg. Real, whole foods will continue to play a prominent, perhaps more prominent, role in this new lifestyle. Remember: We do not limit fat or cholesterol in the Wheat Belly lifestyle because they do not cause heart disease or health problems. They never did, despite the astounding amount of bad science, dietary bungling, and politics that went into promoting that misguided message.

We will also be adding new ingredients that allow you to re-create familiar, grain-based dishes. After all, we still have to contend with children and grandchildren, entertain friends, and enjoy holidays with others, so having an arsenal of healthy replacement ingredients for, say, wheat flour or cornstarch means you can create a delicious cheesecake, birthday cake, or pumpkin pie that everyone (including you) will love. You may not have known that nut meals and flours are wonderful for baking muffins and cupcakes and easily fit into your Wheat Belly lifestyle; they are therefore prominent items in this shopping list. Blueberry muffins and pepperoni pizza, for instance, can be re-created using grain-free ingredients without added sugar.

In addition to the top 10 recipes found in Chapter 9, you will find many more recipes consistent with this lifestyle in *Wheat Belly Cookbook* and *Wheat Belly 30-Minute (or Less!) Cookbook*. If you'll be following the sample 7-day menu plan in Chapter 10, there is another shopping list after the first one below that includes all the ingredients required to make each and every one of the recipes included in the plan.

I've also included some of the basic foods needed to begin adding prebiotic fibers to your diet, to further restore bowel and overall health.

A GENERAL WHEAT BELLY SHOPPING LIST

ALMOND MEAL, ALMOND FLOUR—Almond meal and almond flour are among the most baking-friendly wheat flour replacements. Almond meal is ground from whole almonds with the skin, while almond flour is ground from blanched almonds without the skin. Of our several choices in grain-free flours, almond flour produces the lightest textured end result, useful in making dishes such as cakes and doughnuts. Use the coarser (and less costly) almond meal for everyday uses when a lighter texture is unimportant.

ALMOND MILK, UNSWEETENED—Almond milk is the strained liquid from ground almonds. It is thinner than cow's milk. Look for unsweetened to avoid unnecessary added sugars. If you wish to make your own (which is delicious), puree whole almonds in your food processor or chopper, then strain through cheesecloth, diluting it with water to the desired thickness. Reserve the pulp for baking or thickening sauces.

BANANAS—We use green, unripe bananas, not ripe yellow, in smoothies, yogurts, kefirs, ice cream, and iced coconut milk for their indigestible prebiotic fibers that help cultivate bowel flora that contributes to restoration of health. Because the sugars are in an indigestible form in an unripe banana, they provide nutrition for bowel flora while yielding zero sugar or carbohydrate.

BONES—Bones saved from meats or obtained from the butcher are used for making soups or stocks. Store in the freezer until ready for use.

CAULIFLOWER—Cauliflower is our go-to replacement for mashed potatoes, rice, stuffing, or dressing. A food chopper or food processor will be required.

CHIA SEEDS—Chia's unique capacity to expand when exposed to water makes it a useful addition to baking, for thickening sauces and jams, and for making puddings and mousses. While it cannot be used as a primary flour, it can be added to other flours to create sturdier structure. Add chia to smoothies, yogurts, kefirs, and other dishes for thickness.

CHOCOLATE—100% chocolate, i.e., cocoa without sugar, is an ideal way to add a rich chocolate taste to a dish. Unlike presweetened chocolates, you can determine just how much sweetness you desire. People with dairy sensitivities can also use 100% chocolate to avoid exposure. Dark chocolates with 85% or more cocoa make a great and handy snack.

COCOA POWDER, UNSWEETENED—Unsweetened is the key. Ghirardelli, Scharffenberger, Hershey, and Trader Joes are among widely available brands.

COCONUT FLOUR—Coconut flour is a staple in our grain-free kitchen. It is best added to other flours to create a finer texture and sturdier structure. Avoid using coconut flour as a primary flour, as it generates a heavy, almost inedible end product.

COCONUT MILK—Coconut milk is an all-around useful food, an excellent replacement if you avoid or wish to minimize dairy products. Canned coconut milk is thicker and is therefore great for thickening sauces and as a replacement for sour cream in recipes. Carton varieties are thinner, best anywhere you'd use milk, such as in coffee or in baking when a thinner liquid is needed. Native Forest, Natural Value, and Trader Joe's canned brands are BPA-free. Alternatively, you can make coconut milk in any consistency by grinding down coconut meat with water and straining out the coarse remains. Or heat dried, shredded, or flaked coconut in boiling water for about 3 minutes, then strain it to yield coconut milk.

COCONUT, SHREDDED AND UNSWEETENED; COCONUT FLAKES—Unsweetened coconut is a terrific way to add texture, chewiness, and flavor to breads, muffins, and other baked foods. It's also a great topping for grain-free cakes, cupcakes, and muffins and can be used to make coconut milk (see "Coconut milk" above). Coconut is rich in potassium and fiber.

DRIED FRUIT—Dried apples, apricots, cranberries, currants, blueberries, pears, strawberries, dates, and figs are useful in your grain-free baked products, though only in small quantities to avoid excessive sugar. Always buy unsweetened, as those sweetened with sugar or high-fructose corn syrup present an excessive sugar load. Alternatively, dehydrate fruit yourself and save on costs.

EGGS—If your budget permits, look for organic eggs obtained from pastured chickens. Truly healthy eggs have a deep yellow, orange, or even red-colored yolks, along with richer flavor.

EXTRACTS—Buy almond, coconut, vanilla, lemon, orange, and peppermint extracts, natural only.

FLAXSEEDS—Flaxseeds can be purchased either pre-ground or whole that you grind yourself. They are rich in fiber and linolenic acid (plant-sourced omega-3), and are a versatile replacement flour used most commonly with almond flour. The most baking-friendly are the golden variety, rather than the brown, which has a musty flavor.

FRUCTOOLIGOSACCHARIDES (FOS)—Purchased as a nutritional supplement in powder form, FOS is related to inulin (below), a fiber that provides prebiotic properties for bowel flora health. Use inulin and FOS interchangeably.

GHEE—Ghee is "clarified butter," the oil from butter with the protein solids removed. It is among the least problematic of dairy products, since whey, casein, and lactose have been removed.

INULIN—This is an inexpensive and convenient nutritional supplement in powder form to add prebiotic fructooligosaccharides to smoothies, yogurt, and other foods. FOS fiber (above) is closely related.

NUT AND SEED BUTTERS—Almond butter, peanut butter, cashew butter, and sunflower seed butter can be purchased as pre-ground butters or ground from whole nuts in your food processor, food chopper, or coffee grinder.

NUT MEALS/FLOURS—Almond meal/flour was already discussed above, but also consider pecans, walnuts, hazelnuts, and cashews.

NUTS—Buy raw almonds, pecans, walnuts, pistachios, hazelnuts, Brazil nuts, and macadamias; look for dry-roasted nuts to avoid unhealthy oils, such as hydrogenated cottonseed or hydrogenated soybean oils. Use chopped walnuts or pecans for baking.

OILS—Buy coconut, avocado, walnut, or extra-virgin or extra-light olive oils, or organic butter or ghee.

POTATOES—Raw white (not sweet) potatoes contain indigestible prebiotic fibers nutritious for bowel flora. Cut into small cubes for a salad, reduce to a puree for sauces (don't heat, however) or smoothies, or chop coarsely and add to a smoothie to help cultivate healthy bowel flora.

SEEDS—Raw sunflower, raw pumpkin, sesame, and chia (discussed above). Whole seeds are useful for making non-grain "granola" or to add crunch to cookies and bars. Seeds can also be ground into flours and used in baking. Sesame seed flour, in particular, can be a very baking-friendly seed flour. (Buy bulk, not the small bottles in the spice aisle.)

SHIRATAKI NOODLES—Noodles and pasta replacements made from the flour of the konjac root are safe, posing virtually no carbohydrate challenge, and provide a modest quantity of prebiotic fibers for bowel flora health. Shirataki is usually found in the grocery store refrigerator and packaged in liquid in single-serve bags, not on shelves with pasta. To serve, drain and rinse in a colander (ignore the slightly fishy odor), then boil in a saucepan briefly to warm and drain once again.

SPAGHETTI SQUASH—Baked spaghetti squash makes an excellent non-grain replacement for spaghetti.

SWEETENERS—Best choices are pure liquid stevia, pure powdered stevia, powdered stevia with inulin (not maltodextrin), powdered erythritol, Wheat-Free Market Virtue Sweetener (1:4 sugar replacement and the most concentrated of all premixed powders, made with erythritol and monk fruit), Lakanto (1:1 sugar replacement made with erythritol and monk fruit), Swerve (1:1 sugar replacement made with inulin and erythritol), Truvía (1:2 sugar replacement made with erythritol and rebiana, an isolate of stevia), and xylitol.

ZUCCHINI—Zucchini cut into noodles—what many call zoodles—is best achieved using a spiral cutter such as a Spiralizer, Spirelli, or one of the other devices on the market. It makes a delicious and healthy replacement for grain-based noodles.

A WHEAT BELLY SHOPPING LIST TO FOLLOW THE 7-DAY MENU PLAN

The list seems long, but I included some items that you likely already have in your kitchen, just for the sake of completeness—though I did leave out common herbs and spices and very common foods such as eggs. This list includes the ingredients needed to prepare all the items on the 7-day menu plan. Should you pick and choose among the recipes, then you can, of course, put together your own shopping list.

While not specified in this list, you should also consider making some choice(s) among the benign, natural sweeteners listed above under "Sweeteners."

Almond extract

Almond meal or flour, 32 ounces

Almond milk, unsweetened (or coconut, hemp, or dairy milk)

Apricots, dried

Artichoke hearts, 1 14-ounce can

Asiago cheese, 2 ounces

Basil, fresh or dried

Beef, ground (not lean), 1½ pounds

Bell peppers, 1 red, 1 green

Berries, mixed, fresh or frozen

Broccoli florets, 1 pound

Brussels sprouts, 1 pound

Cauliflower, 2 large heads

Celery, 1 bunch

Cheddar cheese, 9 slices

Cherry tomatoes, 8 ounces

Chicken stock/broth, 4 cups

Chicken thighs, ¼ pound (boneless and skinless, or remove bones and skin)

Chorizo sausage, 6 ounces

Cilantro, fresh

Coconut, shredded, unsweetened

Coconut flour, 12 to 16 ounces

Coconut milk, 4 14-ounce cans (or heavy cream, organic)

Coconut milk, unsweetened (carton; or unsweetened almond, hemp, or dairy milk)

Coconut oil

Cucumber, 1

Eggplant, 2 medium

Feta cheese, 1 cup crumbled

Flaxseeds, ground golden

Ginger, dried and fresh

Green beans, 8 ounces

Green onions, 5 to 6

Ham, precooked, 12 ounces

Ham, sliced, 4 ounces

Hemp milk, unsweetened (or unsweetened almond, coconut, or dairy milk)

Hot sauce, 1 bottle

Kale, 8 ounces, fresh or frozen

Lemon juice, freshly squeezed or bottled

Molasses

Mortadella sausage, 2 ounces

Mozzarella cheese, shredded or whole, 24 ounces

Muffuletta spread or tapenade

Mushrooms, baby bella, 8 ounces

Olives, black or kalamata, pitted, 1 cup

Oregano, fresh or dried

Parmesan cheese, grated

Peanut butter, natural

Pecans

Pepperoni, uncured, 16 ounces

Pinto beans, 1 15-ounce can

Pizza sauce, 1 14-ounce jar—choose brands with the least sugar and no high-fructose corn syrup

Provolone, 4 ounces

Pumpkin seeds, raw

Ricotta cheese, 3 cups

Romano cheese, grated

Sausage, Italian, 8 ounces

Spinach, 4 cups fresh or 1 10-ounce package frozen

Sun-dried tomatoes in olive oil, 1 jar

Sunflower seeds, raw

Sweet potato, 1 medium

Thai fish sauce (or gluten-free soy sauce or tamari)

Tomatoes, diced, 1 14-ounce can

Tomato paste, 1 6-ounce can

Tomato sauce (jar), 2 24-ounce jars (or 2 28-ounce cans whole peeled tomatoes and 6 ounces tomato paste for each jar if you choose to make your own tomato sauce)

Vanilla extract

Walnuts

Zucchini, 4½ pounds

CHAPTER 12

WHEAT BELLY HAPPY HOUR: SAFELY NAVIGATING GRAIN-FREE ALCOHOLIC BEVERAGES

YES, ALCOHOLIC BEVERAGES can indeed fit happily into your Wheat Belly lifestyle. However, you have to be careful to select drinks that you can enjoy but that do not reverse the wonderful health and weight benefits you have achieved.

Understand that while you are actively trying to lose weight, more than one alcoholic drink will shut down your capacity to lose weight that day. Ideally, you should not drink, or you should at least sharply curtail your consumption, while trying to lose weight. Then, once you have achieved your goal weight, loosening up to two drinks per day is perfectly safe (provided you have no history of struggles with alcohol).

In choosing safe alcoholic beverages, we have to be aware of 1) beverages brewed from grains or containing grain-based ingredients, and 2) carbohydrate/sugar content that might be excessive (keep in mind our rule of 15 grams [g] of net carbs per meal, and factor the drink into the meal). Remember: Just because something is grain-free does not always mean it is otherwise without health problems. Jelly beans contain no grains but are not healthy. Alcoholic beverages are no different.

To safely enjoy alcoholic beverages during your health-empowering, weight-loss-achieving Wheat Belly lifestyle, here are your choices.

BEER

Most ales, beers, malt liquors, and lagers are brewed from grains and contain grain proteins that stimulate appetite and inflammation and initiate autoimmunity. People with celiac disease or the most extreme forms of gluten sensitivity should avoid beers altogether except those designated gluten-free; likewise, those of us trying to escape the health effects of grains should avoid these beers.

Gluten-free beers made from sorghum, rice, buckwheat, millet, or chicory are available but tend to be moderate to high in carbohydrate content—more than a single bottle or serving, and you exceed our net carb cutoff. While sorghum, rice, and millet are grains (buckwheat and chicory are not), the low quantity of proteins seems not to provoke reactions in people without extreme gluten sensitivity or allergy.

Among alcoholic beverages, beer is therefore the most hazardous, so be careful. If you must have a beer, among the least problematic are:

BARD'S—Brewed from sorghum without barley, this beer is truly gluten-free. It contains 14.2 g carbohydrate per 12-ounce bottle, so more than one and you exceed our net carb cutoff.

BUD LIGHT AND MICHELOB ULTRA—The Anheuser Busch Bud Light beer is brewed from rice but also contains barley malt, so the most severely gluten-sensitive should not indulge. One 12-ounce bottle contains 6.6 g of carbohydrate. Michelob Ultra is also brewed from rice with barley malt but is even lower in carbohydrates, with 2.6 g per 12-ounce serving.

GREEN'S GLUTEN-FREE BEERS—A UK brewer, Green's provides several gluten-free choices made from sorghum, millet, buckwheat, brown rice, and "deglutenised" barley malt. They are not grain-free and have low quantities of grain proteins. Go carefully here and make judgments based on individual experience. Carbohydrate content of these beers range from 10 to 14 g per 330-milliliter bottle.

REDBRIDGE—Redbridge is brewed from sorghum and, while gluten-free, is still brewed from a grain. Carbohydrate content is high at 16.4 g per bottle; a full 12 ounces exceeds our carb cutoff.

Other choices include:

Glutenator from Epic Brewing Company in Salt Lake City, Utah, is gluten-free with 16 g net carbs per

11 ounces and is brewed from sweet potatoes and molasses.

Omission beers are brewed from malted barley with the gluten removed and are available in an IPA, lager, and ale.

SPIRITS

Spirits are a mixed bag, but you are likely to find at least several that you can safely enjoy. Avoid flavored varieties of vodka or rum, as they are loaded with sugar and/or high-fructose corn syrup. Stick to simple, unflavored spirits such as:

BRANDIES AND COGNACS—Distilled from wine, brandies, cognacs, and Armagnacs are generally safe. Safe cognac brands include Grand Marnier, Courvoisier, and Rémy Martin. There are exceptions, such as Martell, which adds caramel coloring (a potential grain exposure). Safe brandies include Calvados, Christian Brothers, and Korbel.

GINS—Brewed from juniper and other herbs without grains, gins are safe.

LIQUEURS—Because of high sugar content, liqueurs are a problem area. Grain-free choices include Kahlua (dairy), fruit liqueurs like triple sec and Cherry Kijafa, amaretto, and Baileys Irish Cream (dairy), but go lightly due to the sugar.

RUM—Rum is distilled from sugarcane and therefore does not contain residues of grain proteins. The fermentation process converts sugar to alcohol, and the end product should have little to no sugar, but manufacturers will often add sugar to enhance flavor. Brands that have minimal sugar include Bacardi, Captain Morgan, and Brugal.

VODKAS BREWED FROM NON-GRAIN SOURCES— Chopin (potatoes), but outside of North America you will have to ask or examine the bottle for sources (there are wheat and rye vodkas from Chopin); and Cîroc (grapes). Recently, many more vodkas are appearing on the market brewed from grapes, quinoa (not a grain), potatoes, and other non-grain sources.

WHISKEYS AND BOURBONS—Like most beers, whiskeys and bourbons are distilled from rye, barley, wheat, and corn and are thereby potential problem sources. However, given the distillation process, whiskeys typically test below the 20 parts per million limit for gluten that the FDA set as a safe threshold for people with celiac disease and gluten sensitivity. Nonetheless, some people still seem to react to whiskeys distilled from grains. Many popular whiskeys such as Jack Daniels (barley, rye, corn), Jameson (barley), and Bushmills (barley) risk a gluten (gliadin) reaction and should be avoided by anyone with celiac disease or other form of extreme gluten (gliadin) sensitivity. People without extreme sensitivities are likely safe, given the very low quantity of grain proteins.

WINE

Of all alcoholic beverage choices, wine fits most easily into this lifestyle, since it is brewed from grapes, and grains are almost never involved in the wine-making process. The driest (least sweet) wines are best: dry reds such as pinot noir, malbec, merlot, and cabernet sauvignon; dry whites such as pinot gris, chardonnay, and sauvignon blanc. Avoid or minimize sweet wines such as sauternes, ice or dessert wines, and ports to avoid any tangles with blood sugar issues. With champagnes and other bubbly wines, look only for those labeled "brut" or "extra brut," since they contain less sugar, the extra brut being the least sugary; and avoid those labeled "sec" or "doux" as they are too sugary.

Avoid wine coolers as they are typically high in sugar or other unhealthy sweeteners and contain barley malt.

CHAPTER 13

THE TOP 5 REASONS FOR PERSISTENT CRAVINGS

FOLLOW THE WHEAT BELLY lifestyle and you should be miraculously freed of hunger and cravings except when physiologically appropriate, such as after not having eaten anything for 6 to 8 hours or longer. It is common for many of us, for example, to eat breakfast, then have no desire for food until dinner. Or have a healthy lunch at noon, then literally forget to eat dinner. In other words, the incessant, rolling, rumbling hunger that plagues modern people and accounts for aggressive, even angry, food quests disappears and is replaced by experiencing only a soft reminder that it might be nice to eat something in the next few hours.

This happens because you have removed all the appetite-stimulating effects hidden in wheat and grains. Gliadin protein–derived opiate peptides, for instance, that stimulate appetite around the clock are now gone. The high blood sugars that occur after eating wheat and grains due to the highly digestible amylopectin A carbohydrate, followed by low blood sugars that bring feelings of extreme hunger, are all gone. And, as you lose weight by following the Wheat Belly lifestyle, sensitivity to the leptin hormone is restored, the signal that tells you that you have had enough to eat.

You will find that you eat only for sustenance, eating just as much as your body requires to survive and be healthy. You are no longer exposed to the unnatural appetite stimulation that leads to the endless cycle of overeating, gaining weight, and never being truly satisfied—the destructive path that most modern people are trapped in. You will be completely freed from this phenomenon, instead only eating when it is physiologically needed.

If you are following the Wheat Belly lifestyle properly, you should *not* be experiencing inappropriate or nonphysiologic hunger and cravings. You should not be hungry 2 hours after a meal or feel desperate hunger prior to every meal or wake up in the middle of the night craving something. If you *are* experiencing any such feelings, then consider this list of the five most common reasons for having these inappropriate impulses:

1. **You continue to be exposed to wheat or grains.** The Wheat Belly lifestyle is a 100 percent, 7-days-a-week, 24-hours-a-day, no-compromise, and complete wheat- and grain-free lifestyle. Anything short of this will booby-trap your health and weight-loss efforts, just as an alcoholic who sneaks a sip of bourbon every now and then will eventually succumb and be right back at square one. "I'm cutting back," "I eat them

only when there's nothing else," "I have a bad day once a week"—all such excuses will stimulate appetite for days to weeks, often to extreme degrees, not to mention continue to drive inflammation, autoimmune disease, heart disease risk, risk for dementia, and other health issues. And don't forget to examine nutritional supplements, prepared smoothie mixes and other processed foods, and prescription drugs for hidden wheat/grain sources. Even a small exposure of, say, a wheat/grain ingredient in a prepackaged smoothie or protein powder mix can be enough to drive appetite to a surprising degree.

2. **You remain fearful of fat.** Or you've lost the natural impulse to take in adequate quantities of fat because of the misguided low-fat message we've been inundated with these last 40 years. Forget all that advice to limit fat. Eat fat. Buy fatty cuts of meat, never lean; don't trim the fat off meat, eat it; save the grease that remains after you prepare bacon and use it for cooking other foods (store in the refrigerator); and use more organic butter and coconut, olive, avocado, and other healthy, non-grain-sourced oils. Don't count fat grams and don't limit fat or oil portion sizes—just enjoy it. Fats don't make you fat; they make you thin and do not cause heart disease. You will know that you have taken in an adequate amount of fats and oils when you find that you are satisfied with less food, are no longer hungry, and remain that way

for many hours. It also makes you indifferent to the doughnuts at the office or the blueberry muffins at the coffee shop.

3.   **You are limiting calories or portion sizes.** You've got to free yourself of the destructive notion that greater calorie intake causes weight gain, and the idea of "calories in, calories out," and all the other advice that makes you choose smaller portion sizes or push the plate away before you are satisfied. Don't worry about calories and eat until you are satisfied. If you were to count calories on your 100 percent wheat- / grain-free lifestyle, it would indeed be substantially less than it used to be during your wheat- /grain-consuming days because you have removed the gliadin-derived opiate peptides that stimulate appetite. But nobody living the Wheat Belly lifestyle should be counting or limiting calories.

4.   **You are overdoing carbohydrates/sugars.** We live during a time when one-third of people are diabetic, another third are prediabetic, and the remaining third are what I call "pre-pre-diabetic" because of the over-proliferation of carbs/sugars in modern processed foods and the resultant resistance to insulin in people who consume such foods. I see people overdoing carbs/sugars in countless ways: including excessive fruit in their smoothies and protein drinks (not to mention the whey protein that also wildly overstimulates insulin release, blocks weight loss, and

leads to increased food consumption); consuming "gluten-free" foods with cornstarch, rice flour, tapioca starch, and potato flour; "carb-loading" for exercise (an unproductive and destructive practice—see the discussion in *Wheat Belly Total Health* for more about this); clinging to former "healthy" habits like eating bran cereals; and being unaware of the carb content of many foods, such as the 24 grams (g) of net carbs in a ripe, medium-size banana—enough to turn off weight loss, trigger high blood sugars, and magnify appetite when high blood sugar is followed by low blood sugar. Remember, if you limit net carbs to no more than 15 g net per meal, you will be relieved of these effects and get extraordinary control over health and weight.

5. **You have failed to cultivate healthy bowel flora.** Lose the wheat and grains and you remove an enormously disruptive factor in bowel health and bowel flora. But bowel flora does not recover fully on its own, at least not for a long time. This is why we purposefully take steps to cultivate healthy bowel flora, just like planting seeds and nourishing a garden. Failure to do so can mean failure to fully reverse autoimmune conditions, failure to fully reverse type 2 diabetes, failure to fully recover mental/emotional health, failure to reduce long-term risk for diverticular disease and colon cancer, and failure to control appetite and impulse. The Wheat Belly lifestyle therefore includes probiotic supplementation followed

by nourishing healthy microorganisms with a lifelong program of prebiotic fibers. This is not only important to curtail any residual and unnatural food cravings, but also critical for your long-term health. I urge you to not neglect this part of your Wheat Belly lifestyle.

Correct these factors and you return to a natural, "soft" hunger meant to ensure sustenance, nothing more, nothing less—the way it was supposed to be all along until the world got this crazy notion of not just eating grains, but making them the cornerstone of every meal, 7 days a week.

CHAPTER 14

AVOID THESE COMMON MISTAKES ON THE WHEAT BELLY LIFESTYLE

NEWCOMERS TO THE Wheat Belly lifestyle often make the same mistakes over and over again. While all of these issues are discussed in *Wheat Belly*, and even more extensively in *Wheat Belly Total Health* and *Wheat Belly 10-Day Grain Detox*, some people overlook crucial pieces of the message.

To help you avoid common mistakes that can booby-trap both health and your ability to lose weight, here is the list of the most common mistakes people make.

EAT GLUTEN-FREE FOODS. Gluten-free foods made with cornstarch, tapioca starch, potato flour, or rice flour should *never* be used in place of wheat or other gluten sources. This is replacing one problem with another. You already know that two slices of whole wheat bread raises blood sugar higher than 6 teaspoons of table sugar. Know what's worse? Gluten-free foods made with cornstarch, tapioca starch, potato flour, and rice flour—they raise blood sugar higher than *all* other foods, including table sugar, candy, and sugary soft drinks. There is no way to negate the destructive health effects of these gluten-free food ingredients, regardless of claims made by manufacturers. Such foods completely turn off the ability to lose weight, often causing weight *gain*, and take you several steps closer to having diabetes and other health problems.

EAT ORGANIC WHEAT. With or without lipstick, a pig is still a pig. Without herbicides or pesticides, wheat is still wheat. Even worse, it's still likely to be modern high-yield semidwarf wheat, the worst of all. Is organic tobacco healthy to smoke? Of course not. Organic wheat is no better. Remember: The Wheat Belly lifestyle is 100 percent free of all wheat and other grains.

EAT TRADITIONAL STRAINS OF WHEAT. This includes spelt, kamut, red fife, Russian wheat, emmer, and einkorn, older strains of wheat that predate changes introduced by geneticists and agribusiness. These strains are indeed less harmful than modern semidwarf strains, *but they are not harmless*. If I had a cigarette that posed 50 percent less risk of heart disease and cancer compared to conventional cigarettes, would that be safe enough for you? I don't think so, but that's how it goes with these traditional strains of wheat, too: less harmful, *not* harmless.

FIND UNHEALTHY FLOUR SUBSTITUTES. Outside of the terrible mistake of gluten-free flours, people sometimes turn to quinoa, buckwheat, brown rice, wild rice, teff, or millet. While none of these flour alternatives have the potential to trigger autoimmune diseases, mind effects, neurological impairment, psychiatric disease, or gastrointestinal disruption as wheat does, they still send blood sugar sky-high and block weight loss. As with gluten-free flours, don't replace a problem with another problem.

TELL YOURSELF, "A LITTLE BIT WON'T HURT!" A bite of your daughter's birthday cake, a couple of pretzels, a little breading on chicken—avoid it all absolutely, 100 percent, without compromise. This is because even a small exposure can retrigger appetite galore, an effect I call "I ate one cookie and gained 30 pounds," because insatiable appetite can be triggered for *days to weeks*, even after a small exposure. (I have indeed witnessed people regain as much as 30 pounds over a month once this process is reignited.) Worse, any health condition that receded with wheat and grain elimination will recur with even a small reexposure: Migraine headaches will return, the pain of fibromyalgia comes back, and the joint disfigurement of rheumatoid arthritis can recur full-force and persist for *months*. Wheat and grains contain such powerfully toxic components that *any* reexposure is a really bad idea.

MISTAKE GLIADIN-DERIVED OPIATE WITHDRAWAL WITH "NEED." Stop the flow of wheat and you cut off the flow of gliadin protein-derived opiates and thereby experience opiate withdrawal symptoms: nausea, fatigue, depression, and headaches for about 1 week. People will sometimes interpret this unpleasant process to mean that your body somehow must "need" wheat. No, it is an opiate withdrawal that you must get through in order to regain health, just as an alcoholic will have to endure alcohol withdrawal to start the process of being freed of its effects.

REMAIN FEARFUL OF FAT. We reject the "eat more healthy whole grain" message and also reject the "cut your total fat, saturated fat, and cholesterol" arguments that gave birth to overreliance on grains. Many people have a tough time with this, having endured more than 40 years of low-fat messaging and the proliferation of low-fat or nonfat products. If you continue to experience hunger or cravings with wheat and grain elimination, it is your body's signal that you are taking in inadequate quantities of fats and oils. Eat fat: Buy fatty cuts of meat, never lean; eat the fat on pork and beef; eat the dark meat and skin on poultry; save drippings to use for cooking; save bones to boil for soup or stock, and don't skim off the gelatin or fat when it cools; use more organic butter or ghee and more coconut oil; eat more avocados; and eat the yolks in eggs. *Never* buy low-fat or nonfat foods— and I really mean never—because there is simply no reason to have removed the fat in the first place and the manufacturing manipulations made to keep a food palatable make it far more unhealthy. Including plentiful fat in your lifestyle induces satiety and will help push away hunger and cravings and does *not* increase risk for cardiovascular disease.

GET INADEQUATE HYDRATION. When you stop consuming all things wheat, blood insulin levels plummet. This results in water loss. If you lose, say, 5 pounds your first week, 2 or 3 pounds of that total can be water loss. This can leave you dehydrated. Oddly, many people interpret the feelings associated with dehydration as hunger. The solution is not more food, but better hydration. Compensate by hydrating more than usual that first week or so, to avoid becoming lightheaded from low blood pressure and prevent eating to relieve the effect, when the problem is really a lack of water. As salt is also lost in the urine, adding back a mineral-rich form of salt, such as sea salt, can be important. Do so by lightly salting your food.

Succeeding at the Wheat Belly lifestyle is really not that tough. Millions of people are now wheat- and grain-free, and many more millions will join this movement in the future. With it, we are going to witness a dramatic tidal wave of health transformations. So don't botch it up with common mistakes that are truly easy to remedy.

CHAPTER 15

WHEAT BELLY SAFE PACKAGED FOODS

AS YOU KNOW by now, the foods that fit best into your Wheat Belly lifestyle are real, whole, single-ingredient foods like asparagus, salmon, and blueberries, foods that generally do not come with brand names or fancy packaging and are unprocessed. But there will be an occasional need for processed and packaged foods, such as pre-ground almond flour to bake muffins or breads.

Here is a listing of such foods—commercially produced but safe—that have served us well in living the Wheat Belly lifestyle. Note that I only list products that are widely available nationwide. There are also locally or regionally produced foods that you should be aware of; since they will be specific to your locale, they are not listed here.

APPLE CIDER VINEGAR

Bragg Organic Raw, Unfiltered Apple Cider Vinegar

COCONUT MILK (CANNED)

Native Forest Organic Coconut Milk

Natural Value Organic Coconut Milk—In addition to being packaged in a non-BPA can and without a problematic replacement can lining, this coconut milk is organic without added emulsifying agents.

Trader Joe's Organic Coconut Milk—Trader Joe's canned coconut milk is packaged in a BPA-free can and contains no emulsifying agents to disrupt bowel flora.

COCONUT OIL

Kirkland Organic Coconut Oil—Cold-pressed and unrefined, the Costco brand of coconut oil is a safe choice and among the most economical.

Nutiva Organic Coconut Oil

Spectrum Organic Unrefined Virgin Coconut Oil

Trader Joe's Organic Virgin Coconut Oil

DARK CHOCOLATE

Green & Black's Organic Dark Chocolate—The 85% cocoa dark chocolate is organic and made without emulsifiers like soy lecithin. (The 70% cocoa chocolate does contain soy lecithin.)

Lindt dark chocolate—Choices include 70%, 85%, and 90% cocoa chocolates that are low in sugar and free of common emulsifiers typically used in chocolates. (Emulsifying agents have the potential for disrupting the mucous lining of the intestinal tract and thereby disrupting bowel flora.)

DELI MEATS

Boar's Head meats—Boar's Head nationally distributes deli meats (chicken, turkey, beef, ham) that are nitrite-free, sourced from humanely raised animals, and free of other problem ingredients such as growth hormone and antibiotics.

FLAXSEEDS

Bob's Red Mill Organic Raw Whole Golden Flaxseed

Flax USA Organic Golden Flax—An organic variety of ground golden flaxseeds available in big-box stores such as Costco, this is the type of baking-friendly pre-ground flaxseeds that work best in Wheat Belly baking recipes.

FLOURS AND MEALS

Bob's Red Mill almond flour and almond meal—The Bob's Red Mill brand has proven very responsive to the ongoing needs of us grain-free bakers and has come out with several different varieties of almond meals and flours. Most major supermarkets and specialty shops carry this brand.

Trader Joe's Just Almond Meal—This is almond meal ground from whole almonds, skin included, thereby yielding a coarser meal. This is a more economical option when a fine texture is not needed, such as for cookies or scones.

Wheat-Free Market All-Purpose Baking Mix—Wheat-Free Market products are created by following Wheat Belly principles. Its All-Purpose Baking Mix and other products are therefore consistent with this program. It is available online at wheatfreemarket.com.

INULIN

Jarrow Formulas Inulin FOS

NOW Organic Inulin—This is a powdered inulin, a prebiotic fiber that can be added to shakes or smoothies and other dishes.

Vitamin Shoppe Miracle Fiber—Here's another powdered inulin, a prebiotic fiber that can be added to shakes or smoothies and other dishes.

KETCHUP

Full Circle Organic Ketchup

Trader Joe's Organic Ketchup—Trader Joe's is one of the brands of ketchup made without problem ingredients such as high-fructose corn syrup; it's also made with organic ingredients.

Whole Foods Market 365 Organic Tomato Ketchup

NATURAL SWEETENERS

Lakanto—A combination of erythritol and monk fruit that yields a 1:1 replacement for sugar, Lakanto is found in some major supermarkets and specialty stores.

SweetLeaf Stevia—SweetLeaf produces a nice selection of powdered and liquid stevia products that are available nationwide in most major supermarkets and health food and specialty stores.

Swerve sweetener—This combination of inulin and erythritol provides a 1:1 sugar equivalent. It is available in most major supermarkets and specialty stores.

Trader Joe's Organic Stevia Extract (powder), Trader Joe's Organic Liquid Stevia

Wheat-Free Market Virtue Sweetener—This is a combination of monk fruit and erythritol that yields a natural sweetener with four times the sweetness of sugar. That means ¼ cup of Virtue Sweetener provides the same sweetening power as 1 cup of sugar, making it among the most economical of natural sweeteners. It is available online at wheatfreemarket.com.

NUT BUTTERS

Justin's Classic Almond Butter

Trader Joe's Almond Butter

Whole Foods Market 365 Almond Butter

CHAPTER 16

10 RULES FOR EATING SAFELY OUTSIDE THE HOME

EATING OUT AT restaurants, visiting friends and relatives, and attending work and school events should be fun and safe to navigate from this lifestyle—but that is simply not always the case. Taking a few precautions and avoiding some problem areas can keep you on track and prevent the nasty reexposure reactions to grains that can occur, regardless of whether the exposure was intentional or inadvertent.

1. Be selective. You should never, of course, expect a host or hostess to accommodate your personal needs at dinner parties, family get-togethers, or picnics. Instead, choose among the foods that you believe are safe. The only danger comes to those who are severely gluten-sensitive or have severe grain allergies. Even cross-contamination (i.e., a utensil or work surface used to prepare a grain-containing food was also used to prepare

a "grain-free" food) can be harmful. In this case, you can only eat foods safely if the host or restaurant assures you that the proper precautions were taken.

2. If attending an event in someone's home, it is *not* rude to provide advance warning that you have dietary restrictions. Be polite and just say something like, "I don't want you to be insulted if you see me being picky or avoiding dishes, because I know I will become ill if I don't watch what I eat."

3. Avoid going to any event hungry. Instead, eat something before going, so you won't be desperate if there are no grain-free options. Then you can just enjoy seltzer, a glass of wine, nuts, etc., until you can get something safe to eat.

4. Ask for a gluten-free menu at restaurants. Some will have them, some will not. If they do, avoid the gluten-free bread, rolls, pizza, and other replacements. But at least you have some reassurance that ingredients like wheat-based bread crumbs or breading are not used and that efforts were (perhaps) made to avoid cross-contamination of utensils and work surfaces. If there is no gluten-free menu, ask the waitstaff politely whether each dish is gluten-free, meaning no flour or bread crumbs were used in the preparation. (This is not the "official" definition of gluten-free, but works fine for most of us without extreme sensitivities.)

5. Always ask if a meat or other food is breaded. I've made this mistake too often, forgetting that some restaurants will bread just about anything, from asparagus to salmon.

6. Beware of fried foods, as foods that appear to be grain-free, such as French fries, are typically fried in the same oil as, say, fried chicken with a wheat flour breading. The only time fried foods are safe is if a segregated frying apparatus is used. (We should minimize consumption of fried foods, as well, given the high temperature used that introduces unhealthy reactions in the food.)

7. Foods such as burgers, hot dogs, burritos, and tacos that ordinarily come wrapped in a grain-containing bun or shell can nearly always be ordered in a lettuce wrap or simply served without the bun or shell.

8. Dessert is a special problem area, as virtually all dessert dishes contain wheat flour and a load of sugar. The only dessert that I find most restaurants will accommodate is a request for fresh berries or fruit with whipped cream. Of course, you could also opt for an after-dinner liqueur, such as cognac, but there is little else to safely choose from. Instead, have a delicious slice of cheesecake when you return home that you made yourself without problem ingredients.

9. In restaurants in which a language barrier may be present—e.g., Chinese, Thai, Korean—look for foods

that are obviously without grains. This reduces your options considerably, typically to only stir-fried veggies or simple meats without sauces, and no rice or anything fried, breaded, or "sweet and sour" (a land mine of sweeteners). If you have the opportunity, frequent a particular restaurant so that you get to know the menu and staff, thereby reducing the hazards of an inadvertent exposure. Those of you with severe gluten sensitivities and/or allergies to grain components should *not* take the chance and should avoid any place in which it is not crystal clear that your foods are gluten-free.

10. If you order a meal but have to skip a grain-containing side dish, such as onion rings or french fries cross-contaminated in shared frying oil, ask that they be replaced with something safe, such as a vegetable side or a side salad.

Local restaurants sometimes make the effort to segregate a gluten-free portion of their kitchen, separating utensils, work surfaces, and grills, but most do not—although they will still declare this-or-that dish to be "gluten-free" just because it was not prepared with a gluten-containing ingredient. If you are among the exceptionally gluten-sensitive, then it pays to have your server make the distinction to avoid unintended exposures. Sadly, at this moment, most restaurants cannot assure absolutely gluten-free food preparation because of nonsegregated use of fryers and grills, for instance, used to prepare grain-containing foods.

Ask questions, be firm, but be courteous. Don't feel obliged to educate restaurant staff; just be clear that this is not a silly request you are making, but one made for health. Don't allow anyone to belittle your concerns with comments like "Oh, you just have a gluten allergy?" or "I think it will be okay. A little bit won't hurt, right?" Take such dismissals as a lack of interest in your concerns and think twice about ordering any dish. Thankfully, you can still succeed in having many delicious and problem-free meals outside the home with just a bit of effort.

SOME SAFE CHAIN RESTAURANT OPTIONS

National chain restaurants—because they have a corporate structure in which decisions can be made centrally and handed down—are more likely to have gluten-free menus or at least choices of dishes that do not contain wheat and grains. Among them are:

APPLEBEE'S—Applebee's has an extensive grilled menu: chicken, steak, and shrimp with various sides or on top of a salad. Most of these are safe, provided you don't eat any bread served on the side. Ask that no breaded meats be used and avoid obvious other grain exposures such as croutons, onion rings, or chow mein noodles. Sauces are another problem area; consult this chart provided by the chain for the safety of its sauces: applebees.com/~/media/

docs/Applebees_Allergen_Info.pdf. The barbecue sauces are safe. However, be aware that just because a sauce does not contain wheat or gluten does not mean it is healthy, as most of these sauces are very sweet and high in sugar. So go carefully and consume as little of the sweet sauce as possible, or ask to have it left off the dish. Also, be aware that these foods are safe for most of us just avoiding wheat and grains, but not safe for those with extreme gluten sensitivities.

THE CHEESECAKE FACTORY—I've eaten dozens of times at Cheesecake Factories around the country and have never been inadvertently exposed to wheat or grains. With its huge menu, you are sure to find a few, if not several, dishes that fit into your tastes and are grain-free. As with all large, busy kitchens, dishes labeled "gluten-free" may or may not be truly gluten-free, so anyone with an exquisite sensitivity should remain vigilant and inquire about the situation in the kitchen. Among safe entrées I've had are Grilled Pork Chop, Grilled Rib-Eye Steak, Jamaican Black Pepper Shrimp (just pass on the rice), Herb Crusted Filet of Salmon, Seared Tuna Tataki Salad, and Fresh Vegetable Salad, as well as the majority of the omelets. Sadly, none of the cheesecakes fit into our lifestyle (though some have consumed only the filling without the crust on the Low Carb Cheesecake without problems, accepting that the sweetener used is bowel flora-disrupting sucralose).

CHILI'S—The Chili's chain does a good job of listing all the allergen information on its Web site: chilis.com/en/locationspecificpdf/menupdf/001.005.0000/chilis allergen generic.pdf. Foods that are free of peanuts, dairy, and other allergens, as well as wheat and gluten, are listed. Among safe choices are: Ancho Chile Salmon, Avocado Sirloin, and Grilled Chicken Salad from the "Fresh Tex Lighter Choices"; Fresh Tex Baby Back Ribs and Steaks; and Caribbean, Fresco, and Santa Fe Chicken Salads. Burgers ordered without the bun and without onion rings or French fries sides are also safe. As with other chain restaurants, however, there are no efforts made to avoid cross-contamination, so the Chili's menu is not safe for the exceptionally gluten-sensitive.

OLIVE GARDEN—Olive Garden has its cooks change gloves and utensils when a gluten-free order comes through, although fryers and grills are not segregated and still risk cross-contamination. Nonetheless, for those of us not among the exceptionally gluten-sensitive, a handful (not many, given that it is largely a pasta restaurant) of safe items are on the menu. They include: Tuscan Sirloin, Herb-Grilled Salmon, and Our Famous House Salad (minus croutons). There are gluten-free rotini pasta dishes available but, as we have discussed, gluten-free pastas are something we absolutely avoid.

RUBY TUESDAY—The grilled meats are safe here as entrées or on top of salads. Among the choices are a variety of steaks and ribs, Grilled Salmon, Jumbo Skewered Shrimp, and Blackened Tilapia. The Grilled Chicken and Grilled Salmon Caesar Salads are safe minus the croutons. There is also a large salad bar that can be easily navigated with plenty of choices. However, as with other restaurants, cross-contamination from utensils, work surfaces, fryers, and grills remain an issue. Allergen information is listed on its Web site: gipsee.com/rubytallergen/Prefs.aspx

FAST FOOD

In general, minimize reliance on fast-food restaurants, as too many ingredient compromises are made to reduce costs or increase palatability or for other reasons, which introduce plenty of processed ingredient land mines. However, there are some chains that you can go to in a pinch and come out grain-unscathed. Some fast-food chains have grain-free options, and many now list allergens on their Web sites (nuts, soy, etc., as well as wheat and gluten). As with most other restaurants, though, none have dedicated gluten-free areas and utensils, so they are not safe for the extremely gluten-sensitive.

CHIPOTLE—You can navigate a safe lunch at Chipotle by getting meats, salads, beans, cheese, salsas, sauces, guacamole, and toppings and avoiding the tacos, burritos, and shells. Allergen information is listed online at https://chipotle.com/allergens.

JIMMY JOHNS—All of this sandwich restaurant's choices are available as Unwiches, which wrap conventional sandwich ingredients in lettuce instead of bread. Note that the same utensils and work surfaces are used to make conventional sandwiches, so cross-contamination is virtually guaranteed here.

PANERA BREAD—Despite the name, Panera actually has some confidently grain-free items on the menu. Because grain figures so prominently in its menu, cross-contamination is virtually guaranteed. Most of us not among the exceptionally sensitive can do fine here with choices such as Green Goddess Cobb Salad with Chicken, Romaine and Kale Caesar Salad with Chicken, and Seasonal Greens Salad. When they offer to include bread or a roll, ask to replace it with an apple or other fruit. Avoid the soups as they are thickened with cornstarch.

QDOBA—As with Chipotle, you can pick and choose your safe ingredients, but just avoid the tacos, burritos, and shells. Allergen information is listed on its Web site: qdoba.com/downloads/Qdoba_Allergen_Info.pdf.

CHAPTER 17

RECOGNIZE HIDDEN
SOURCES OF WHEAT
AND CORN

GRAINS COME IN an incredible variety of forms, often hidden as additives, thickeners, or coatings. The colorful names can fool you into thinking that no wheat is present: Couscous, matzoh, orzo, graham, farro, panko, and bran, for example, are all wheat.

Be aware of the potential for cross-contamination, i.e., potential grain contamination from utensils, work surfaces, airborne particles, or liquids. This is most problematic for people with extreme gluten sensitivities or allergy to a grain component. If a food is labeled "gluten-free," then it should have been prepared in a facility where cross-contamination would *not* have occurred. Potential for cross-contamination is especially tricky in restaurants; very few have the ability to avoid cross-contamination, though an increasing number are taking on the challenge as the market for these foods grows.

To qualify as "gluten-free" according to FDA criteria,

products must be both free of gluten and produced in a gluten-free facility to prevent cross-contamination. The FDA's cutoff for qualifying as "gluten-free" is no more than 20 parts per million (ppm). This means that, for the seriously sensitive, even an ingredient label that does not list wheat or any buzzwords for wheat—such as "modified food starch"—can still contain some quantity of gluten. When in doubt, contact the product's customer service department to inquire whether a gluten-free facility was used.

Note that wheat-free does not equate with gluten-free in food labeling. Wheat-free can mean, for instance, that barley malt or rye is used in place of wheat, but both are sources of gluten and other grain-sourced contaminants. Also note that many medications and nutritional supplements contain wheat or corn. Check with your pharmacist or check the medication's package insert and check the label on supplements. If a prescription drug contains a wheat and/or corn derivative, consult your doctor for an alternative.

Here are some not-so-obvious ways that foods can contain wheat. A question mark (?) following an item means it is either variable or uncertain (given the manufacturers' reluctance or inability to specify the source).

HIDDEN SOURCES OF WHEAT

Baguette

Beignet

Bran

Brioche

Bulgur

Burrito

Caramel coloring (?)

Caramel flavoring (?)

Couscous

Crepe

Croutons

Dextrimaltose

Durum

Einkorn

Emmer

Emulsifiers

Farina

Farro

Focaccia

Fu (gluten in Asian foods)

Gnocchi

Graham flour

Gravy

Hydrolyzed vegetable protein

Hydrolyzed wheat starch

Kamut

Maltodextrin

Matzo

Modified food starch (?)

Orzo

Panko (a bread crumb mixture used in Japanese cooking)

Ramen

Roux (wheat-based sauce or thickener)

Rusk

Rye

Seitan (nearly pure gluten used in place of meat)

Semolina

Soba (mostly buckwheat but usually also includes wheat)

Spelt

Stabilizers

Strudel

Tabbouleh

Tart

Textured vegetable protein (?)

Triticale

Triticum

Udon

Vital wheat gluten

Wheat bran

Wheat germ

Wraps

HIDDEN SOURCES OF CORN

One of the difficulties with corn products is that there are literally hundreds of common food ingredients derived from corn—such as dextrose, dextrin, maltodextrin, high-fructose corn syrup, fructose, maltitol, polydextrose, ethanol, caramel coloring, and artificial flavorings—that will not be identified as being corn-sourced. However, the process to generate these products from corn reduces protein content to negligible levels, and they are therefore generally not a problem for grain exposure for the majority (though these products, especially sugars, pose other problems of their own). By adhering to the general Wheat Belly rule of avoiding most processed foods, you will handily avoid most of the hidden sources of corn.

Baking powder

Chewing gum

Corn chips

Corn oil

Corn sweetener

Grits

High-fructose corn syrup

Hominy

Hydrolyzed corn protein

Hydrolyzed cornstarch

Maize

Mixed vegetable oil, vegetable oil

Modified corn starch

Modified food starch

Polenta

Popcorn

Succotash

Taco shells

Vegetable chips

Vegetable oil

CONCLUSION

CUT CALORIES AND you might—might—lose a few pounds while having to battle constant hunger. Cut fat and eat low-fat or nonfat foods and you will likewise endure increased cravings for junk carbohydrates to compensate for lost calories, while experiencing all manner of health problems, from irritable bowel syndrome to high blood sugars and cholesterol.

But banish all wheat and grains from your life and incredible things happen, typically far beyond your wildest expectations. Not only does weight drop, often precipitously and without hunger, but after the initial withdrawal/detoxification fireworks are over, you experience clearer thinking without mind "fog," increased energy, receding joint and muscle discomfort, and reversal of many cases of fibromyalgia, migraine headaches, and autoimmune diseases. Blood sugar plummets so much that people on insulin or other diabetes medications have to reduce or eliminate medications. Blood pressure drops such that hypertension prescriptions likewise have to be reduced or eliminated. The majority of people with acid reflux and irritable bowel syndrome are freed of symptoms within the first week. Literally hundreds of health conditions can recede beginning within days of undertaking this process.

In other words, the Wheat Belly lifestyle is not just a program to shed a few pounds or fit back into a size 4 dress. It is a program that restores health in a breathtaking number of ways, resulting in weight loss because excess weight is just one visible manifestation of health and diet gone wrong. Renewed health therefore shows itself as weight loss, but also as healthier skin, more youthful energy, and remarks from friends and family that you look 10 or 20 years younger.

What you carry in your hands in *Wheat Belly Slim Guide* is part of the solution to so many health and weight problems that you may have thought were simply the product of prior bad habits, bad genes, or just bad luck, but were really the product of a world given the wrong message about diet. Get the message right, put it to work using simple tools like this guide, and you will be back on course to reclaim a level of health, slenderness, and youthful vigor that you may have thought were beyond reach.

I invite you to share your experiences—successes, hurdles, questions, photos, recipes—on Wheat Belly social media, especially the official Wheat Belly Facebook page and the Wheat Belly blog.

INDEX